The Theory and Treatment of Fevers

You are holding a reproduction of an original work that is in the public domain in the United States of America, and possibly other countries. You may freely copy and distribute this work as no entity (individual or corporate) has a copyright on the body of the work. This book may contain prior copyright references, and library stamps (as most of these works were scanned from library copies). These have been scanned and retained as part of the historical artifact.

This book may have occasional imperfections such as missing or blurred pages, poor pictures, errant marks, etc. that were either part of the original artifact, or were introduced by the scanning process. We believe this work is culturally important, and despite the imperfections, have elected to bring it back into print as part of our continuing commitment to the preservation of printed works worldwide. We appreciate your understanding of the imperfections in the preservation process, and hope you enjoy this valuable book.

THE
THEORY AND TREATMENT
OF
FEVERS,

BY

DR. JOHN SAPPINGTON,

SALINE COUNTY, MISSOURI.

REVISED AND CORRECTED

BY FERDINANDO STITH, M.D.,

FRANKLIN, TENNESSEE.

A Paul may plant, an Apollos may water, but the increase is of God.—*First Epist. Paul to the Cor., Chap. 3d, 6th verse.*

ARROW ROCK:
PUBLISHED BY THE AUTHOR.
1844.

MISSOURI DISTRICT, ss.

Be it remembered, that on the 28th day of October, A. D. one thousand eight hundred and forty-three, John Sappington, of said District, hath deposited in this office the title of a book, the right whereof he claims as proprietor, in the words and figures following, to wit: "The Theory and Treatment of Fevers, by Dr. John Sappington, of Saline County, Missouri." In conformity with an act of Congress entitled an act to amend the several acts respecting copy-rights.

I, Jason Harrison, Clerk of the United States' District Court for the District of Missouri, do certify, that the above and foregoing is a true copy of the original of record in my office. In testimony whereof, I have hereunto set my hand and affixed the [SEAL.] seal of said court at my office, in the city of Jefferson, the 28th day of October, 1843. JASON HARRISON, Clerk.

Entered, according to the act of Congress, in the year one thousand eight hundred and forty-three, by Dr. John Sappington, in the clerk's office of the district court of the United States for the Missouri district.

J. Fagan, Stereotyper.
T. K. & P. G. Collins, Printers.

RECOMMENDATIONS.

The author has thought fit to lay before the reader the following only, out of the many statements that he might have published in support of his practice.

From Gen. T. A. Smith, Brigadier General in the Army of the United States, and formerly Receiver of Public Moneys at Franklin, Missouri:

I have been personally and intimately acquainted with Dr. John Sappington, of Saline county, Missouri, for more than twenty years, and have no hesitation in saying, that he has as much reputation as a physician as any man. He stands pre-eminent in the treatment of fevers. From what I have seen of him, and heard from others, he has ever been a warm and zealous advocate for the early and free use of sudorifics, tonics, and stimulants.

T. A. SMITH.

From the Hon. R. W. Wells, United States District Judge for the State of Missouri:

City of Jefferson, January 25, 1841.

Dr. John Sappington,

Sir—I have heard with much pleasure, that you intend publishing a work on the treatment and cure of fevers. I hope it will not be abandoned. For many years, as you know, I have been desirous you should prepare and publish such a work, believing it would be a public benefit. On my own personal knowledge, I declare that your treatment of fevers has been most eminently successful, whilst it is my deliberate opinion—an opinion formed on twenty years of observation and experience in this State—that the constant and excessive use of calomel, so common during all that time, has generally been injurious in the particular cases, and the fruitful cause of broken constitutions and a train of awful diseases and consequent suffering. If you succeed in preventing the excessive and general use of calomel, you will deserve a statue of gold to be erected by the mothers of Missouri.

Wishing your work great success, I remain your friend and servant.

R. W. WELLS.

RECOMMENDATIONS.

We the undersigned, citizens of Saline county, in the State of Missouri, having understood that Dr. John Sappington, of this county, is about to publish a work, entitled "Sappington on Fevers," consider it to be our duty, both to the doctor and to the public, to state the facts connected with our knowledge of him both as a man and physician.

We, therefore, take great pleasure in saying, that as a man, he stands as fair as any one—that he commands the confidence and respect of all who know him. And, as a physician, more especially in the treatment of fevers, he stands unrivalled in his profession, and the proof of this fact is to be found in his services having been sought after far and near, during the time he continued to practise medicine, and we doubt not, if his bodily infirmity from old age would allow him now to continue the practice of his profession, that it would be the same case yet.

D. PULLIAM,
JNO. A. TRIGG,
WM. L. DURRETT,
BERNIS BROWN,
JOSEPH FIELD,
WYATT BINGHAM,
A. TRIGG,
CORNELIUS DAVIS,
O. B. PEARSON,
C. W. DAVIS,
HENRY NAVE,
JOHN B. GROVE,
ISAAC NEFF,
WM. T. BROWN,
EDMUND BROWN,
JAMES HARRIS,
SAMUEL GROVE,
WM. N. OLIVER,
WILLIAM L. ISH,
RICHARD DURRETT,
JESSE ROMINE,
WILLIAM LEWIS,
JOHN PIPER,
HENRY KELTER,
JACOB ISH,
NATHAN HOLLIWAY.

I, Robert Field, Sheriff of Saline county, do hereby certify that the persons whose names are above subscribed, signed the same in my presence. That they are all old settlers in our county, and men of the first respectability and standing.

Given under my hand this 29th June, 1843.

ROBERT FIELD.

STATE OF MISSOURI, } To wit:
County of Saline,

I, John A. Trigg, Clerk of the Circuit Court for the county aforesaid, do hereby certify, that Robert Field, whose name is above subscribed, is the Sheriff of Saline county, for witness whereof I have [SEAL.] hereunto set my hand and affixed the seal of said Court, the 5th day of July, 1843.

JNO. A. TRIGG, Clerk.

As Dr. John Sappington, of Saline county, Missouri, is about to publish a treatise on fevers, and as we, some of the citizens of Howard county, in said State of Missouri, whose names are hereunto

RECOMMENDATIONS. v

subscribed, many of whom have been acquainted with him for twenty years, feel it a duty we owe him, and more particularly a duty we owe to the community at a distance, that his character and standing should be made known. As a man he is much respected and highly esteemed; as a physician he stood at the head of the profession as long as he was able to ride and practise medicine; his services were sought for far and near, and no doubt would still be but for his bodily infirmity from old age.

ARCH'D WOODS,	H. L. BOON,
A. F. WALDEN,	NATHANIEL FORD
CHARLES CANOLE,	GRAY BYNUM,
JOHN JACKSON,	JOHN W. PRICE,
DAVID WORKMAN,	RICHARD G. CRIGLAR.
W. BUSTER,	JOHN ROOKER,
JOHN P. MORRIS,	URIEL SEBREE,
JOHN KING,	JOSEPH SEARS,
WILLIAM WARD,	JOHN B. CLARK,
J. KINGSBURY,	ROBERT BROWN,
W. MOROWS,	ROBERT HANCOCK,
WILLIAM MUNRO,	JO. DAVIS,
JAMES MUNRO,	ROBERT COOPER,
JAMES TURDAN,	BENJAMIN WATTS,
JOEL PREWITT,	WILLIAM BOTTS,
E. R. PULLIAM,	JAMES JACKSON, Sen.,
GEORGE CHAPMAN,	HARRISON STAPLETON.

I, Lewis Criglar, Sheriff of Howard county, in the State of Missouri, do hereby certify that the gentlemen whose names appear to the foregoing instrument of writing, are all personally known to me to be the identical persons which their names represent, who made their signatures in my presence, and are all gentlemen of acknowledged worth, intelligence and respectability.

Given under my hand at Fayette, this 27th day of September 1841. LEWIS CRIGLAR, Sheriff H. C.

STATE OF MISSOURI, }
County of Howard, } To wit:

I, Gray Bynum, Clerk of the Circuit Court within and for the county of Howard, in the State of Missouri, do hereby certify that Lewis Criglar, whose certificate appears above, is personally known to me to be the real person who subscribed said certificate, and that he subscribed his name thereto in my presence, for the purpose therein mentioned, and that he is, and was at the time of subscribing the same, the acting Sheriff of said county, and that as an officer and a man the standing and character of Mr. Criglar are both equally above reproach. In testimony whereof I have hereto signed my name and
[SEAL.] affixed the seal of said Court at my office, in the town of Fayette, in said county, this 27th day of September, 1841.
GRAY BYNUM, Clerk,
By S. BYNUM, D. C.

RECOMMENDATIONS.

OAKLAND, HOWARD COUNTY, MO.,
April 5th, 1841.

Dr. John Sappington,

Dear Sir—In reply to the information you have communicated to me, of an intention you have to publish a treatise on fevers, I take pleasure in having it in my power to state, that I have known you as a practising physician for more than fifteen years, in which time we have had frequent occasions of meeting, and consulting each other in the chamber of febrile patients, especially in protracted cases, proceeding from marsh and similar miasmata. I esteem it but right, that I should say to you, I have been long since impressed with the belief in those cases that your judgment, in the exhibition of sudorifics, tonics, and stimulants, in regard to time, and quantity, is superior to most of our most reputable physicians. I, at least, am sure that you have commenced their use with good effect, at a stage of fever, when I would have entered upon them with much hesitation and doubt.

Believe me, dear sir, to remain with esteem, your friend,
SAMUEL T. CREWS, M. D.

AT HOME, HOWARD COUNTY, MO.,
June 9th, 1841.

Dr. John Sappington:

When I had the pleasure of an interview with you, sometime since, I promised to transmit you a few lines relative to my opinion concerning your course of the practice of medicine in fevers.

From an acquaintance of upwards of twenty years, and occasionally during that time, having occasion to be in consultation with you in critical cases of fever, I could not but observe in your treatment, *the free and early use of sudorifics, tonics, and stimulants.*

This practice was used by you sooner than my notions of practice indicated. It is but sheer justice to add my humble testimony to the common fame of your success in the practice. I can therefore with propriety say, that but few men in this country have practised with more success in fevers than yourself.

I will, however, take this occasion to add, that in what very appropriately in this State is called *congestive bilious fever,* I could not, nor cannot now, treat it successfully *without the lancet and calomel!* Your friend,

JOHN J. LOWRY.

We, the undersigned citizens of Cooper county, and State of Missouri, having been long and well acquainted with the character and standing of Dr. John Sappington, of Saline county, and State aforesaid, do hereby certify that, in our opinion, as a man and gentleman, none stand fairer; and, as a physician, he ranks at the head of his profession, and is universally regarded as pre-eminent in the treatment of fevers in their various forms. The above is given that the public abroad may know the character of a man who we understand will publish a Book on Fevers. Given under our hands in the year 1843.

ROBERT WALLACE, GEO. W. MORTEN,
JNO. M'CUTCHEN,   JAS. M. MAJOR,
WM. SHIELDS,   BENJ. WATKINS SHARP.
B. EMMONS FERRY, JOHN MILLER,
I. LIONBURGER,   JAMES COLE,
CHAS. CHILTON,   JOHN S. M'FARLAND,
JAMES CARTER,   ALLEN PORTER,
A. R. RHOADS,   A. W. CROUTHER,
JAMES HILL,   JOHN I. KELLY,
ABRAHAM BARNES,   ROBERT POGUE,
ABRAHAM H. NEAL, I. S. ANDERSON,
PETER PIERCE,   ED. B. M'PHERSON.
ISAIAH THOMAS,

This is to certify that all persons whose names are subscribed to the foregoing certificate are resident citizens of the county of Cooper, in the State of Missouri.

Given from under my hand this 15th day of November, 1843.

ISAAC LIONBURGER,
Sheriff of Cooper county, Missouri.

STATE OF MISSOURI, } SS.
County of Cooper, }

I, B. Emmons Ferry, Clerk of the County Court within and for the county aforesaid, do hereby certify that Isaac Lionburger, Esq., whose name is subscribed to the foregoing certificate, is, and was at the date of said certificate, acting Sheriff of the county aforesaid, regularly commissioned and qualified as such, and that his acts in the premises are entitled to full faith and credit. In testimony whereof I, the Clerk aforesaid, have hereunto set my hand and seal of office, at the city of Boonville this 15th day of November, A. D., 1843.

B. EMMONS FERRY, Clerk.

STATE OF TENNESSEE, 1843.

The undersigned take great pleasure in giving their certificates, being called on to do so, to and in favour of Dr. John Sappington's Anti-Fever Pills, as being the best, the most successful and valuable pills in the cure and treatment of fevers in their various forms and grades that they have ever witnessed, and their knowledge is derived from a long and intimate knowledge, having had and seen them tested for many years past.

They have won favour and a name, as is shown by their extensive use, when or wherever they have been used; are far above the other remedies of the day in their peculiar adaptation to the cure of fevers.

Given under our hands and seals, the date above.

JAMES STEELE,
J. R. BLEDSOE,
THOMAS SIMMONS,
SIMMONDS & BYLES, Red Mound, Tenn.
WILLIAM B. HALL, Lawrenceburg, Tenn.
M. L. SMITH, Humphrey's county, Tenn.
J. H. K. WYLY, Camden, Tenn.
J. W. GRIZZARD, Huntingdon, Tenn.
RANDALL ROBINSON, Locust Grove, Tenn.
M. D. FURR, Dyersburgh, Tenn.

STATE OF TENNESSEE, 1843.

We, the undersigned, having had Dr. John Sappington's Anti-Fever Pills for sale for several years past, do hereby knowingly certify, that we believe them to be the best, the most successful and valuable medicine in the treatment and cure of fevers, in their various forms and aspects, that has ever before been offered to the public.

We have known intricate cases of fever cured by their use, when all other remedies had failed. The increased demand for them, when and wherever there is sickness, for many years past, and their extensive sale throughout the country, show in what high repute they stand in the communities in which they are and have been used as a remedial agent in the cure of fevers.

Given under our hands and seals the year above written,

WILLIAM S. WISDOM, Purdy, Tennessee.
W. B. FERRY, Jack's Creek, Tenn.
REDDICK DISHOUGH, Hardeman co., Tenn.
WILLIAM WASHAM, Giles county, Tenn.
ALFRED JETT, Montgomery county, Tenn.
W. G. WYNN, Onward, Stewart co., Tenn.
Z. NOELL, Henry county, Tenn.
J. M. GILBERT, Weakley county, Tenn.
W. LANDRUM & CO., Dresden, Tenn.

STATE OF ALABAMA, 1843.

The undersigned are of opinion, that in the cure and treatment of fevers, both intermittent, bilious, or any other form of fever, Dr.

RECOMMENDATIONS.

John Sappington's Anti-Fever Pills come as near a specific as any other medicines they have ever known used. This belief is derived from a long acquaintance with their use in our respective sections of country, and from having used ourselves, and seen others use them. Their great and deserved popularity sustains us in the assertion, that as a remedial agent in the cure and general treatment of fevers they are not surpassed, if equalled by any other mode or treatment, that we have ever witnessed.

Given under our hands and seals this year above written.

   FRANKLIN ARMSTRONG.
   J. W. COWLING, Lowndes county.
   JAMES K. WHITMAN, Lowndesboro, Ala.
   JAMES GREENWOOD, Benton, Lowndes co.
   JOHN R. SOMMERVILLE, Benton, Lowndes co.
   THOMAS J. WATTS, Mt. Willing, Lowndes co.
   JEREMIAH WATTS, do.   do.
   JOHN BARGE, Barge's, Butler co., Ala.
   JACOB RALL, Monroeville, Ala.
   W. B. ANDREWS, Burnsville, Dallas co.
   T. H. HAMPTON, Havanna, Green county.
   JOHN LITTLE, Tuscaloosa, Ala.

           STATE OF ALABAMA, 1843.

We, the undersigned, from a long and an intimate acquaintance both from having used ourselves, and seen others use it, in our respective sections of country, do believe that Dr. John Sappington's Anti-Fever Pills are the nearest a sovereign remedy in the cure and treatment of fevers in their various forms, than that of any other we have ever witnessed, or than any other ever offered to the public. They stand far above the other remedies of the day, in our State, as is shown by their almost universal use, for the past several years, and their increased demand yearly.

Given under our hands and seals. the date above.

   VANCE & BEIGHT, Russelville, Franklin co.
   THA. WALKER, Macon county, Ala.
   LEVI LINDSEY, Sen., Fayette C. H., Ala.
   WILLIAM CLIFTON, Fayette county, Ala.
   S. B. COBB, Fayette county, Ala.
   SAMUEL LINTON, Pickens county, Ala.
   WILLIAM CHALMERS, do.   do.
   NABES & CHALMERS, Carrolton, Pickens co.
   JOHN T. GARDNER, Bridgeville, Ala.
   JOHN COCHRAN, Cochran's Mills, Ala.
   JOSEPH KING, Pickens county, Ala.
   T. H. GODDEN, Marion, Perry county, Ala.

RECOMMENDATIONS.

WILLIAM D. JONES, Sumter county, Ala.
SAMUEL WILLIAMS, Sumter county, Ala.
PHILEMON KIRKLAND, Greene county, Ala.
ADDISON FIKE, Clinton, Ala.
MOSES HUBBARD, Springfield, Ala.
HANNA & TRAVIS, Greene county, Ala.
STEPHEN HEARON, Choctaw Corner, Clarke co.
JOHN W. FIGURES, Coffeeville, Clarke co.
JAMES SAVAGE, Macon county, Ala.
JOHN W. G. FOSTER, Claiborne county, Ala.
E. J. JOHNSON, Prairie Bluff, Ala.
JOHN PATTERSON, Prairieville, Marengo co.

UNION SPRINGS, MACON CO., ALA.
September, 1841.

Dear Sir—Chance, during the present year, has thrown in my way some of your fever pills, and from a small experiment I have made with them, I am enabled to say they answer a better purpose in arresting intermittent and remittent fever than any medicine, or combination of medicines, I have ever used. I have for several years been engaged in the practice of physic, and can truly say that your pills appear to fill a vacuum in the treatment of those maladies which all my reading and experience has heretofore failed to supply, and I candidly believe they are entitled to a preference over all other medicines or mode of treatment known to the profession.

I have always sought the most ready means for the relief of suffering humanity, and believe it may be found in your pills. I should be glad to use them extensively in my practice, but know of no chance I have to procure them; neither do I know if you are in the habit of furnishing them to physicians. If you are, and can put me on a footing to get some, I should be glad to be supplied with some one hundred boxes. This place is fifty miles east of Montgomery, Ala., and about the same distance southwest of Columbus, Ga. I would take some on commission, and use every means of giving them notoriety in parts where their virtue is not known, or otherwise would be glad to buy some to use in practice.

A line from you would be thankfully received. Direct to this place.

Respectfully, your obedient servant,
J. B. COLEMAN.

N. B. Should it be convenient, you can send me some of the above pills to the care of T. B. Costor, Druggist, Montgomery, Alabama; to whom also I refer you for information about myself.
J. B. C.

RECOMMENDATIONS.

GREENSBORO, ALA., May 23, 1843.

Dr. John Sappington:

Dear Sir—I have been in the annual use of your celebrated Anti-Fever Pills for the last seven years, during which time I have had opportunities of using them in every variety of fevers, from their first inception or mildest form to the most aggravated form of bilious fever, wherein they have many times, to my utter astonishment, proved surprisingly effectual, and I have almost invariably administered them with the happiest effects. Therefore I feel no hesitancy in recommending them to the community as a safe remedy in all febrile diseases.

I am yours with respect,

DANIEL EDDINS.

TUSCALOOSA, ALA., May 24, 1843.

Dr. John Sappington:

Dear Sir—For several years last past I have sold from my drug-store many hundred boxes of your Anti-Fever Pills, and have in no case known them fail to produce the desired effect, when used according to your prescription.

I have also used them in my practice with equal success. In a word, I consider them a most valuable medicine in fevers.

Yours, respectfully,

SAMUEL M. MEEK.

TERRE HAUTE, IND., August 15, 1843.

Dr. John Sappington:

Dear Sir—I have known your pills to be used in fevers for several years past, and from what I have seen of their effects, and heard from others who have used them in the cure of fevers, I consider them superior to any of the preparations heretofore before the public. Respectfully yours,

J. F. KING.

PATOKA, GIBSON Co., IND., Sept. 10, 1843.

Dr. John Sappington:

Dear Sir—Having used your pills in my family for several years past, and having sold several hundred boxes of them in this and the adjoining counties, I freely say, their effect in the cure of fevers and ague and fever, has been most happy and prompt. Those who buy the pills speak well of them. In short, I never *knew* or *heard* of a *single* failure where the directions were fully followed.

Respectfully yours, WILLIAM FRENCH.

RECOMMENDATIONS.

VINCENNES, IND., Oct. 14, 1843.

Dr John Sappington:

Dear Sir—An extensive acquaintance in the State of Indiana has enabled us to hear much said of your valuable pills in the cure of fevers. We can, therefore, unhesitatingly state that they are generally considered the best remedy for fevers that has been offered to the people.

**HARRISON B. SHEPHERD, ANDREW BERRY,
ABRAHAM SMITH,   SAML. EMISON.
A. B. DANIEL,**

WHITE PIGEON, MICH., Sept. 21, 1843.

Dr. John Sappington:

Dear Sir—In this State your Anti-Fever Pills for the last few years have gained a name for themselves of unequalled popularity for the cure of all descriptions of fevers, when properly applied.

Your obedient servant,   H. M'ARTHUR.

FLORENCE, MICH., Oct. 12, 1843.

Dr. John Sappington:

Dear Sir—I have had your Anti-Fever Pills for sale a number of years; they have now a name deservedly great for the cure of fevers, and are decidedly the most popular remedy of the day in their peculiar adaptation for the successful cure of fevers.

JOHN HOWARD.

PIQUA, OHIO, January 1, 1844.

Dr. John Sappington

Dear Sir—Having been agent for the sale of your valuable Anti-Fever Pills for several years past, it affords me pleasure to be able to state that out of more than five hundred cases, as I believe, where I have witnessed their effects, in my own family as well as amongst my relatives and acquaintances, they have proved, in, I believe, ninety-nine cases out of one hundred, a most salutary remedy. So great is my confidence in their efficacy, that I would not now hesitate to warrant a cure of the ague and fever from their use in 1000 cases for 25 cents a case. I have resided in the Miami Valley for nearly 40 years, some 13 or 14 of which I have been engaged in the drug business; I have used, and seen used, almost all the medicines that are in use in the United States, and have no hesitation in saying that I believe Sappington's Pills to be the best ague medicine in the world. Yours, very respectfully,

M. G. MITCHELL.

DEDICATION.

To the people of the United States, more particularly that portion of them, with whom I have had a personal acquaintance, and from whom I have always received a cordial welcome and generous support; and also to all that portion of the medical profession, who can so far divest themselves of the prejudice of education as to give to the following pages an unbiassed and impartial perusal, is this work inscribed by its author.

PREFACE.

At the present era of the world, in proportion as mental illumination is advancing in the different portions ot the earth, just so is the opinion becoming prevalent, that that individual who renders the greatest service to the human family is entitled to the highest honours.

History informs us that warriors, statesmen, and philosophers have ever been justly regarded as competitors for the highest distinctions, and the greatest honours. And although the summit heights of usefulness cannot be reached by all, still this consideration should not discourage the rest of mankind from doing whatever may be in their power to ameliorate the sufferings, and better the condition of the human race.

It has been our lot to toil in that department of human investigation, which has for its especial object the prevention and the cure of all those ills that necessarily arise out of the frailties and imperfections inherent in the physical organization of man.

Now he who advances the just knowledge of his physical nature, and a knowledge of the modifying powers of any of the physical agents that act on his varied sensibilities and impressibilities, we consider as achieving an important step in the science of human happiness.

The author of this work has not the vanity to believe, nor does he wish it to be understood, that he considers himself as having claims above all others upon the great mass of mankind for anything that he has done, or that he may do. Yet he cannot resist the impression that the treatise which he now presents to the public will be found, upon a fair trial, to contain the most certain, speedy, and effectual plan, for the cure of fevers, that has hitherto been offered to the public.

As this treatise is designed more for the benefit of the public than the profession, the author has studiously endeavoured to avoid technicalities, and to present it in the most simple and plain language that he could possibly employ, so that every reader may clearly and fully understand and comprehend his views on every subject that he may treat.

This work will be found to differ from the theories and practice of the present time, and indeed from all that have preceded it, upon the nature and treatment of fevers.

For whilst almost every physician is of opinion that the different forms of fever are dissimilar in their nature from the beginning, and that notwithstanding this dissimilarity in them, that they all have a more or less inflammatory tendency, the author of this work believes them to depend upon a uniform law of nature, which establishes a unity of disease, in accordance with the unity of vitality, and that they have their origin and progress in debility.

While the larger number of physicians consider depletion, either by bleeding, puking, or purging, or by the use of nauseating medicines, and sometimes by all of these means combined, as indispensably necessary for the cure of fevers, the author has limited their use very much, disapproves of their use entirely in the last stages, and relies almost exclusively on tonics and their auxiliaries to effect the same desirable object.

He also believes that all pukes and purgatives are irritants and not stimulants, and that fever proper is a disease of irritation, and that it never runs up into active inflammation. He likewise believes that the Peruvian bark or quinine is a tonic, and not a stimulant, as is generally supposed.

Although he was himself trained to the theory and practice of medicine as commonly taught in the schools in the days of his pupilage, and in part imbibed them, yet the result of his observation and experience, in an extensive practice for nearly fifty years, has fully satisfied him of the great superiority of this practice, over that of either the depletory or the stimulant.

For while this plan of treatment effects a speedy and more certain cure without prostration, the two systems hat are based upon opposite extremes often prolong disease and suffering. Or if a cure be effected at all, it is done in despite of such treatment, and not unfrequently so impairing the constitution, that the unfortunate being remains an invalid throughout the balance of his life.

The author is well aware of the responsibility he has assumed in daring to offer to the public a work of this kind, differing as it does from all published opinions on the theory and treatment of fevers. He is also aware of the unkind feelings it will probably excite among the medical profession towards him.

While he continued to ride and to practise medicine he was often accused of empiricism, because he dared to differ from a theory and practice that has been impressed on their minds, and the minds of the community as orthodox; and when, too, in justification of his practice, he in the main supported the same physiological doctrines that they themselves did, and now do, as will appear in the body of this work.

He thinks he might say, without doing them injustice, or without having any unkind feelings for them as men, that there are very many of them, who, (no matter what a man's acquirements or success in practice might be) if he dared to differ from them, or from their favourite leaders in the schools, would either treat him with cold, silent contempt, or attempt slily to defame his character.

This seems to be the effect of deep-rooted feelings, probably based on natural organization, and, I suppose, being regarded as the result of fixed prime causes and the circumstances of education, ought therefore to be excused.

But the author, knowing the success of his practice from his own experience and observation, contrasted with that of any other, fully justifies himself in the opinion, that he hazards nothing as a man, or as a physician, in asserting that it is the safest, most speedy, and successful practice extant for the cure of fevers.

This opinion is further confirmed by the unexampled success attending the administration of his Anti-Fever Pills throughout a large portion of the United States, both North and South, for the last eight or ten years.

He, therefore, considers himself called upon to present both his theory and practice to the public in the manner that he has adopted, in order to afford them a full and fair opportunity of testing it for themselves, and by their decision is he willing to stand or fall.

CONTENTS.

	PAGE
Preface,	15
Chapter I.—The author's reasons why he has departed from the practice of the old school physicians, and all others, in the treatment and cure of fevers,	21
Chapter II.—A short outline of the animal economy,	29
Chapter III.—The author's views and opinions in relation to the inconsistency and irrationality of attempting to cure fevers principally by depletion,	51
Chapter IV.—The author's practice and treatment in the cure of fevers,	76
Chapter V.—The author's views on the subject of the unity of fevers,	85
Chapter VI.—Of intermittent, or ague and fever,	92
Chapter VII.—Of common bilious, or bilious-remittent fever,	99
Chapter VIII.—Cholera infantum,	112
Chapter IX.—Yellow fever,	118
Chapter X.—Influenza,	146
Chapter XI.—Of mild typhus, or nervous fever,	148
Chapter XII.—Of cold plague, or spotted fever,	156
Chapter XIII.—Of scarlet fever,	164
Chapter XIV.—Of measles,	170
Chapter XV.—Of child-bed or puerperal fever,	176
Chapter XVI.—An alphabetical arrangement of the classes of medicines used in this work,	182
Appendix,	206
Report of a case of stone in the bladder,	207
Remarks on Asiatic cholera,	212

THEORY AND TREATMENT

OF

FEVERS.

CHAPTER FIRST.

The opinion has been long since entertained, and by some eminent medical philosophers expressed, that a theory founded upon nature, a theory "that should bind together the scattered facts of medical knowledge, and converge into one point of view the laws of organic life, would thus on many accounts contribute to the interest of society. It would capacitate men of moderate abilities to practise the art of healing with real advantage to the public; it would enable every one of literary acquirements to distinguish the genuine disciples of medicine from those of boastful effrontery or of wily address; and would teach mankind in some important situations the *knowledge of themselves.*"—Darwin's Zoonomia.

As I have long since departed from the theory and practice in which I was principally taught, and am now engaged in writing against them, it may be proper that I should give my reasons to the public for so doing.

I commenced the study of medicine about the time that Cullin and Rush, at the head of their respective schools, were lecturing and promulgating to the world their views on blood-letting and other modes of depletion, then adopted by the followers of the depletive or anti-phlogistic theories. I was instructed in those doctrines, and after having practised with my preceptor for about five years, who was a scientific and experienced practitioner, and who was inclined to the Brunonian and Darwinian doctrines, using tonics and stimulants earlier and more generally than was common, I entered on the duties of my profession on my own responsibility, and was at least as successful as those around me.

But not being satisfied with the result of my own practice, and less so with that of others, which was chiefly that of bleeding and acting on the stomach and bowels with emetics and cathartics, as long as we thought the patients could bear them; then treating the case principally with what we called cooling anti-phlogistic medicines, and which indeed was of little or no use, until the patients died, or recovered by the mere sanative operations of the constitution. After having practised medicine several years, and having undergone a considerable change in my views and opinions relative to the nature and character of some diseases and some remedies, I attended a course of medical lectures in the University at Philadelphia, where I became confirmed in the opinion that I was reasonably acquainted with the different theories and practices of the day, but which only served to confirm me of their error in very many particulars.

It is a serious evil in society and much to be regretted, that the ruling or dominant party in medicine, like that of bigots in religion, are always willing to wage an exterminating warfare against any theory or practice that is new, or that differs from their views of propriety, without investigating the principles upon which it is based, or knowing the result of the practice in scarcely any way whatever.

Being aware of this fact, and believing that I had made a valuable discovery in medicine, or that I had more fully developed the properties of an article of the Materia Medica that had long been in use, but was still very imperfectly understood, I was unwilling that it should be lost to society.

I therefore prepared and sent forth to the public large quantities of my Anti-Fever Pills, and at the same time concealing their composition that they might acquire a reputation upon their own intrinsic worth.

Now that the virtue of these pills to the amount of at least one million of boxes has been tested by the people of the United States, and of the Republic of Texas, and up to this date have maintained an improving reputation; thereby sustaining the correctness of my theory, for the mystery is not more in the drug than in the use I have made of it; I presume that the public will begin to see how strangely and unjustly the medicinal properties of the Peruvian bark and its preparations have been perverted, and that instead of its being injurious when taken in the hot stage of fevers, as has been frequently said of it, it is not only entirely safe and beneficial in that or any other stage, but it is the best febrifuge, tonic and antiseptic known.

The truth of my position is still further maintained by the facts, that since the distribution of my anti-fever pills (now ten years or more) announcing the facts that their virtues resided in their tonic properties, and further that they did not contain any arsenic, many apothecaries and physicians have endeavoured to imitate them, and have vended the same or some similar tonic remedies to be used in all stages of fever.

Now when I had established the fact that tonics might with safety and with efficacy be used in all fevers, it was not a difficult task for practitioners to select the particular drug best calculated to meet the indications, hence all of them no doubt have had more or less of quinine in their nostrums. I am led to these remarks from an apprehension that so soon as these pages shall be presented to the public eye, that the practitioners of medicine and the venders of fever nostrums may not attempt to harass the public mind by refusing to acknowledge the fact, that quinine or some other vegetable tonic constituted the basis of their specifics for fever.

Not long after I commenced the practice of medicine, an old pamphlet fell into my hands giving an account of the accidental discovery of the medicinal properties of the Peruvian bark, which was to the best of my recollection as follows:

A sect of religious persons, known by the name of Jesuits, in their intercourse with the inhabitants of South America, in passing through the province of Peru, were necessitated to drink and to use for cooking the waters of certain ponds on their way. The water in some of these ponds was strongly impregnated with the properties of the bark of certain trees that grew in or around them.

Other ponds in their route which had none of those trees in or about them, were in like manner resorted to for water.

Those persons who happened to fall sick at the latter ponds, either died or remained there until the tardy efforts of nature and a good constitution enabled them so far to recover of their illness as to continue their journey; while but few of those persons who became sick of fevers at the former ponds, where the trees grew, and who were compelled to use for all purposes the water of these ponds, were rarely detained more than a few days before they were cured, and enabled to pursue their journey.

This fact became so notorious, the cases of cure so numerous, that it caused much enquiry and investigation; when it was ascertained satisfactorily that these cures were effected by the water, in consequence of its being impregnated with the medicinal property of the bark of these trees. Hence the first knowledge that we have of the bark of these trees, is under the name of Jesuit's, or Peruvian bark.

Many of these unfortunate people were stricken down, at various times, by fever; and in that hot climate it is reasonable to suppose that many were of the lowest grade and most malignant character.

It is said there was a time when the Peruvian bark (not the sulphate of quinine) sold for its own weight in gold, which is a proof of its once esteemed value.

Since my knowledge of medicine, the best quality of bark has sold in Philadelphia at from five to ten dollars per pound. But, for the last twenty-five or thirty years, it has varied from fifty cents to a dollar per pound. From these facts we might infer that the use of it had been very much restricted in that short space of time, and that calomel, and other poisonous and prostrating medicines, had been substituted in its stead.

Although I read this account given of the bark in the pamphlet, with much interest and a good share of faith,—although I had myself experienced the good effects of it in the height of fevers,—yet it was some years before I could entirely rid myself of the prejudice which I had acquired against it.

Many times have I sat by the bedside of my patients for days together, giving it, anxiously waiting to see the effect it would have upon them; at the same time amusing their minds, and the minds of their attendants, by giving some placebo that I knew to be harmless and useless. I found no increased heat in the skin, no increased thirst, no increased arterial action, nor any other aggravated symptom, that I could ascribe to the bark.

On the contrary, in a few hours, or a few days at most, the skin would become soft and moist; or perhaps a free and generous flow of perspiration would ensue, the thirst abate, the fretful and irritated condition of the pulse would moderate, and the feverish heat and restless anxiety (always more or less attendant on fevers) subside, in much less time than by any other course of treatment I had ever seen, and the patients recover their health more speedily, and with less prostration or debility.

I have taken the bark myself, (in good health—for mere experiment,) in ounce doses, which is equal to ten or twelve grains of quinine, and although it produced some dizziness or swimming in the head, there was no increased heat in the skin, or increased action in the pulse.

I presume that it acts more directly on the brain and the nervous system, but produces no such effects as an over-portion of intoxicating liquors, or the preparations of opium do, nor does languor or prostration follow as a natural consequence, as is the case with the use of stimulants proper.

We think it more than probable that the bark would never have lost the reputation it promised to obtain at the time of its first introduction, if we had then known, as we now do, how to separate its active medicinal properties from its cortical and inert matter. The irritating and supposed stimulating effects ascribed to it by the older practitioners, may, in our opinions, be more justly assignable to its bulk, and the presence of the cortical matter with which it was encumbered, than to its salt, in which modern chemistry has shown its virtues to reside.

Before the improved condition and highly concentrated preparation of the bark, in the form of quinine, was known, I was, on many occasions, much inconvenienced, and sometimes defeated in getting as much taken as I wished.

Partly owing to the prejudices of the people, causing them to fear that it would increase their fevers, and partly to the fact that, in some instances, the stomach would not retain it, or that it would pass off on the bowels as a purgative,—in either event my object was more or less defeated.

The names of Pelletier and Caventou, who first separated the pure alkaline salt, called quina, from the bulky and inert mass in which nature had placed it, deserve to be remembered with gratitude by all mankind.

Since that fortunate era in medicine, I have been enabled to administer the bark at any stage, and in any quantities that I might think advisable, without fear of injury to my patients, or exciting any fear in their minds. This discovery has not only afforded me heart-felt gratification,—for the reason that it enabled me to give more prompt and certain relief to the sick,—but it has been instrumental in giving to me a character and standing in my profession, well calculated to excite the envy of the physicians around me. But this I desired not; for I did not conceal from them, in our consultations, my views on either the theory or practice which gave me such superior success. It seemed that the most melancholy experience was not sufficient to convince them of their errors, and they still, from the mere force of education, considered my practice as empirical.

Far be it from us to censure any one for tenaciously adhering to the prejudices of education, however erroneous such prejudices may be; let the Jew be Jew still—let the Rushite be Rushite: for we deem it a wise provision in the economy of nature to have it thus. We only seek to apologize for the course that we, as individual laborers in the cause of humanity, have pursued.

Every philosophic mind must know that all innovations have to work their way to popular favor on their own intrinsic merits. The discovery of truth is alike open to all men: it is the exclusive property of no one—it is a part of the eternal bounty of nature, and was, from the beginning, designed for all. Then let all seek, and let no one be debarred the privilege of proclaiming whatever he may have found.

We are well aware of the necessity and the importance of well-endowed, well-regulated establishments, for the purposes of mental, moral and manual discipline, in every department of human thought, and of human action.

We know, also, that one of the marked characteristics, one of the marked advantages of civilization, consists in the division of labor. Such division tends, unquestionably, to the perfection of science, and to the perfection of skill in the manipulations of the arts.

Hence, in the earlier periods of the world,—as we see from the records of Egyptian, of Babylonian, Grecian, Roman, and other historians,—resulted the establishment under state authorities; the laws of castes, of trades, of professions, and of privileged orders in society.

Now, such laws, such regulations, such usages, may have been rendered necessary at those epochs of time, from the nature of the elements of humanity then under progress of development. But it is easy to trace in the downfall of those states the deleterious influence of castes, and of chartered privileges, and protection upon the various branches of human occupancy. In proportion as trades and professions are fostered by law, in the same proportion do their votaries become indolent, and the wholesome spirit of emulation dies away.

The check thus given to the freedom of thought, causes the spirit, the true science of law, divinity, medicine and the arts, to dwindle, to lose its vitality, and the minds of men to become fixed, and, as it were, stereotyped into settled formularies.

We have been led into the preceding train of thought from the manifestations given by many of the states of this union, in their legislative enactments, chartering, either directly or indirectly, sectarian colleges calculated to foster partisan religionists.

Also laws entitled acts to regulate the practice of medicine; many of these contrary to the spirit of this government, and calculated to promote the interest of a particular class, to the detriment of others.

The effect of the one is to fetter, to stagnate the advancement of the study of the spiritual nature and the spiritual happiness of man; while that of the other retards the progressive knowledge of the laws of his physical nature, and the true mode of improving his condition, his happiness, as based in his physical nature and influenced by physical causes.

What better evidence could be desired of the error and the selfishness of all these petitions and petitioners for protection, than the universal fact that they sprung from the professions, and not from the people whose welfare they hypocritically profess to guard and serve.

" 'Tis strange! 'tis passing strange!" at this enlightened day, at this half rational era of the world; in this free, this new, this self-created republic; that the people, the true, the only legitimate sovereigns of the earth, should not know what they needed, what they wanted, what they desired, what was best for them, as well as the self-styled guardians of their bodies and their souls.

We do not wish to be understood as finding fault with, or objecting to, any thing that now is, or that has transpired. O'er the past and the present man has no control. Whatever has been, has been; whatever is, is; and whether right or wrong, we cannot change it. Let us, then, gather lessons of wisdom from a knowledge of the present and the past, by which to direct our own future destinies, over which alone an indulgent Providence has willed to man a modifying influence.

CHAPTER II.

CONTAINING A BRIEF OUTLINE OF THE ANIMAL ECONOMY.

That the general reader may have some idea of the offices of some of the most important organs of the human system, and that members of the profession may conceive more readily of the manner in which I suppose diseases are contracted, and the most natural and speedy way by which they may be cured, I deem it proper that I should give a short account of the functions of those organs which are supposed to be mostly involved in fevers, as well as most other diseases.

It is the office of the stomach to receive all the ingesta, both solid and fluid, designed for the nourishment and growth of the whole body. It is by the very peculiar action of this organ and its secretions that the first process, an important part of digestion, is performed.

So soon as the stomach shall have performed its office on the varied aliments and drinks taken in, then the whole of the residual mass passes on to the first portion of the intestinal canal, called the duodenum, where the ingesta in its present state of preparation comes in contact with the peculiar fluids secreted by the liver and the pancreas, called bile, and pancreatic juice. Through the agency of these secretions is the nutritious matter called chyle supposed to be elaborated from the food; and now the lacteals and absorbents situated in this particular portion of the canal, stimulated by its presence, take it up to carry it into the general circulation for the nourishment and the support of the whole body.

The digestion being thus principally performed by the stomach and duodenum, the food continues its passage downwards through the remaining small and large intestines, to make its exit from the bowels by stool; being no longer fit for the purposes of the economy; however, affording more or less matter for the absorbents throughout its whole extent.

The lacteals and absorbents above-mentioned having carried the nutritious portion of that which was taken into the stomach, the chyle, into the receptacle of the chyle, where, assuming a white or milky appearance, it is carried through this duct to be emptied into the left subclavian vein, at or near its junction with the internal jugular, and there mixing with the venous blood, is carried into the great descending vein called vena cava; from thence into the two cavities of the heart, (the right auricle and the right ventricle,) from which latter it is propelled into the pulmonary arteries, and carried by the various ramifications of the same through the lungs, in which it is properly prepared by the action of the air for the subsequent uses of the system. Being thus assimilated, it is carried back by the pulmonary veins to the left auricle, from thence to the left ventricle, and from thence it is propelled into the great artery on the spine called aorta, and from thence is distributed through its numerous branches to every part of the body. Having passed through this routine of elaboration and circulation, and attained its highest state of vitality, it reaches its final destination in the capillary tissues, the fine net-work to be found in the parenchymæ of all the glands, as well as all the surfaces, both internal and external, called surfaces of relation, the most considerable of which is the external cutaneous surface.

Now the objects to be accomplished in the animal economy by the circulation of the blood (which has been justly called the vital fluid) are manifold: but for our present purposes it will only be necessary to dwell on two of them; the one is the deposition of atomic molecules,—in other words, nutrition,—the other is the performance of the offices of depuration, or the elimination of useless or redundant matter from the system. In this latter capacity the skin and its auxiliary, the lungs, by their respective processes of sensible and insensible perspiration, and halitus, or exhalations, have duties assigned them more extended, and equally important and imperious, as any of the functions of the whole animal economy.

That portion of the blood not expended or eliminated in the capillaries, is returned to the heart and lungs for further preparation, or retained and preserved in the circulation for the future wants of the economy, and not returned to the stomach and bowels, where it was first received and where it was first elaborated.

It has been long since demonstrated by many physiologists, that there is more recrementitious matter cast off through the pores of the skin, and by its auxiliary, the lungs, (for these surfaces, in point of depuration, perform very analogous offices,) than by stool, by urine, and by all the other outlets of the human body united. This fact should never be lost sight of, for on it rests an important step toward the knowledge and treatment of disease.

There are many persons, individuals who enjoy good health,—usually of good digestion, too,—the exhalations from whose bodies partake of the fœtor of the excrementitious matter of the bowels. There are others, again, whose perspiration has a decided urinous odor. In such persons, perspiration is usually abundant; while their healthy habits are, to urinate but little, and to defecate but seldom.

It should be recollected that every organ of the body,—the liver, the lungs, the kidneys, the stomach, the bowels, the brain, the nerves, the muscles, et cetera,—all receive their support by and through the before-mentioned processes of digestion, circulation and assimilation; and that all of these organs perform their respective offices promptly and harmoniously when under the influence of their appropriate stimuli, and when not obstructed or deranged by some offending cause or causes. But these causes are numerous in kind, character and quality, as also variable in degree.

We come, now, to the investigation of that portion of the animal structure called the encephalon, or brain, and its appendages, or elongations, the nerves. Here we find both structural and functional phenomena not merely peculiar, but, in many respects, widely varying from that of all other organs, yet, like other portions of organic matter, inseparably connected with and dependent on other organs, other structures, for its support—particularly that of the vascular and muscular systems.

The one peculiarity of the brain consists in its exemption from cellular reticular tissues and the deposits of adipose matter,* the intermittent character of its functions, and the functions of the nervous system generally, as is evinced by the imperious necessity of sleep, while other functions of animal life are in full force—such as circulation, respiration, digestion, et cetera. Another peculiarity consists in its susceptibility of being acted on, and that in a very eminent degree, by the instrumentality of moral and intellectual stimuli, as well as physical stimuli, which, alone, make an impression on all other organs. It is to this latter peculiarity that we wish to draw the attention of medical men; its uses and its influences we think much more extensive and important than is generally supposed by the members of the profession. We do not mean to enter into any enquiries upon the spiritual or immaterial agencies in human phenomena; but shall consider the brain in a strictly natural and philosophic light, as the seat of all the sensations, passions and emotions, and as the material organ of thought.

It is by the instrumentality of this organ, through the medium of its nerves, that all sense of pleasure or of pain is felt—that aversion or desire is produced; that every organ is made alive to its appropriate stimuli; and every muscle in the body would be deprived of motion or sensation without its benign influence. It exerts, therefore, an all-pervading power, both in sickness and in health.

---

* The brain, though not affording adipose matter (in its common sense,) is furnished with peculiar fatty acids, containing phosphorus.

The animal machine is not governed by the laws of mechanics; nor by those of hydraulics; nor those of chemistry; nor by a union of them all: but by laws, by forces, peculiar to vegetable and animal existences, called laws of vitality, and which are more or less modified by the influences of the before-named laws or powers, as we shall endeavor to explain. The mechanic laws are recognized, and most aptly exemplified in the bony and muscular structures, in their aptitudes to the purposes for which they were designed, and in the amenability of the whole, both solids and fluids, to the powers of gravitation. The hydraulic laws are observable, to a limited extent, in the valvular structure, so common throughout the vascular and lymphatic systems; and the influence of both must be admitted from the comfort and advantages of position, more especially the advantages of the recumbent position during sleep, thereby giving rest to the solids, while it facilitates the passage of the fluid elements through the whole body.

As to chemical laws, we conceive them to play still a much more important part in vital machinery. Physiologists and chemists have both long since concurred in the general belief that the oxygen of the atmosphere, and the function of respiration, had a decided agency in the production of animal heat; however widely they may have differed in their particular views as to the *modus operandi* in producing that effect.

Whoever desires to keep pace with the progressive developments of organic chemistry, will be pleased with the recent experiments of Professor Leibig, of Germany, contained in his reports on organic chemistry, applied to physiology and pathology. The learned professor has gone into a careful analysis of every portion of the human body, then into the analysis of every description of aliment, both fluid and solid, on which he lives, that he might discover all those elements in our food best suited to the production of the elements necessary for the body. The results to which he has arrived are truly interesting, some of which we beg leave to introduce. He says:—"That every motion, every manifestation of force, is the result of the transformation of the structure, or of its substance; every conception, every mental affection, is followed by changes in the chemical nature of the secreted fluids.

"Every thought, every sensation is accompanied by a change in the composition of the substance of the brain It is to supply the waste thus produced that food is necessary. Again, vitality is the ruling agent by which the chemical powers are made to subserve its purposes; but the acting forces are chemical."

The professor further observes: "That the mutual action between the elements of food and the oxygen of the air is the source of animal heat. All living creatures, whose existence depends on the absorption of oxygen, possess within themselves a source of heat independent of the medium in which they exist."

This heat, in Professor Leibig's opinion, is wholly due to the combustion of the carbon and hydrogen contained in the food which they consume.

To this last result of the professor we are not entirely ready to give our assent, unless he intends to include the galvanic and electric agency in the development of caloric, as coming under his views of the union of oxygen and carbon, or oxygen and hydrogen, and in this way account for the sudden developments of heat which we frequently witness under the impressions of moral causes; such as the sudden flush of modesty on the virgin's cheek, which we think to be too instantaneous to be achieved through the heart and the circulation.

Another very remarkable and useful result to which the professor's experiments have led, is the connexion between the food on which we live, and the physiologica results to the economy. From all the articles of die which man is accustomed to consume, he has been enabled to point out those that abound most in the elements for the formation of bone, of muscle, of fat, of cerebral mass, or even the matter of heat; or, in other words, the diet to give strength of bone, of muscle, of passion and of thought, or which abounds in the elements of heat.

So important a part does the phenomenon of chemico-animal heat perform in the animal economy, that some deluded minds have been simple enough to contend that heat is life; that the want of it is death: they mistake a symptom, a single phenomenon for the summum totum. Perfect life, perfect health, consists not in the high degree of elevation of temperature; but in the ability to maintain a proper degree under different circumstances, and that degree is different in the different orders of animated nature.

What should we say of all those numerous families of insects, of reptiles, yea, of the whole round of cold-blooded creatures, that for the most part remain torpid, cold, and, even in many instances, frozen through the whole winter; but yet revive again with the return of the genial heat of spring? Shall we pronounce them dead! or in a state of suspended animation merely?

That the general reader may the better comprehend our theme, and that our own particular views may be more fully carried home to their understandings, we propose, in the next place, to give as concise and as clear an account of the theories of medicine that have at various periods of the world found favor in human estimation, as the nature of the subject and the nature of this work will permit. Engaged as we are in efforts to cast what light we can on a particular class of diseases only, we do not feel ourselves under any obligation to make a critical examination of the history of medicine; or even to sum up in regular order a classification of the varied chains of thought that have at different times occupied the minds of distinguished professors and writers; but to introduce and dwell on such only as have obtained the greatest notoriety, and such as may best suit our own present purposes.

What, then, should we understand by the science of medicine? It is that science which treats of diseases and their remedies. The term medicina, from the verb medior, to heal, has given to the profession the title of the healing art: with the Greeks it was mostly confined to surgery and to the use of external remedies. It was for Hippocrates to lay the foundation on which all succeeding ages and nations have built. He first separated it from philosophy, gave it the form of a distinct science, and personally observed the progress of diseases, as well as the effects of remedies: on this account he is styled the inventor of the medicina clinica.

But we are endeavouring to lift the veil of mystery from that feature in the physiognomy of man called fever. Now, the theory of fever is inseparable from the theory of medicine, which comprises the doctrines of the nature of man, the nature of his diseases and their remedies; and this involves the doctrines of vitality, the laws of human life,—and these again the will of Deity as made manifest in man; in other words, the theology of humanity.

Now man, since his first introduction on this theatre, has been ever subjected to great and perpetual changes; every condition of his existence stamps its peculiar character on his physiognomy, and with it corresponding moral and mental manifestations; he is the subject of continued change; he is modified by climate, by soil, by food; and even by the face of the country in which he lives. To use the language of V. Cousin, " man changes much; man changes often; yet he changes not radically." On these facts is based the usefulness of history, whether it be of law, medicine, or divinity. The absolute truths of humanity, ever the same, in proportion as they become disengaged from the masses of error with which they are by nature encumbered, are destined to flow on from generation to generation, from nation to nation, in one continued stream of light, in ceaseless and rapid augmentation to the end of time; or to the terminus of all human truths, the full unfolding of man to man; the complete development of the philosophy of humanity.

The preceding route of inquiry has been crowded with votaries now more than two thousand years; and though the labors of no one individual have been entirely crowned with success, the world is still much indebted to every one for his particular toils; for, while in the distance of time and the darkness of ignorance that overshadowed the earth any light was better than no light, and the many lights enabled the latest laborers to compound light, and thereby obtain a clearer and a brighter view than fell to the lot of any of his individual predecessors. To what particular position in this department of philosophy, this immense and complicated circuit of ideas, we may have reached, wil be for posterity to decide.

That the terminus has not yet been reached is certain from the fact that none has stood the test of time and of criticism, not one has carried conviction to the minds of all, however lauded, however popular many for a season may have been. It seems that we ever have been, and still are, in a state of progression; and progression itself implies a position short of maturity.

All absolute, disembodied, disencumbered, spiritualized truths, are pure elements of philosophy, from whatever source they may spring. Law, medicine, religion, fashions, are the subjects of continued change, because they partake of the changeableness of man, while the pure elements of truth which belong to them are the same to-day, yesterday and forever.

But let us return to Hippocrates, the Coan sage: He was a philosopher who turned his attention to medicine as one of its branches. Now, all that portion of him which has withstood the test of time belongs to the philosophic element of which he was composed, or contains the particular truths of the science of medicine disencumbered by himself, as we shall presently show.

Philosophy was anterior to medicine; it is coeval with man, with theology. Now, theology and philosophy when rightly understood, are one and the same thing. It was, it is, it ever will be, a prime, a constant, a universal want, a universal desire of humanity; while medicine and law are only secondary and accidental wants.

Medicine, as a science, commenced with the Coan sage. Anteriorly all things were under the dominion of theocracy and the state. But in proportion as time rolled on, population increased, wants multiplied, and the minds of men agitated in the cradle of civilization, the ancient dynasties gave way, then from the elements of humanity sprang the professions, commonly called the learned professions, of law, medicine and divinity. These assuming the guardianship of the people and the state, branched off each in separate tracks, to pursue its destined course; all professing, and with more or less sincerity too, to be laborers in the cause of human good. Each, still standing apart, has continued its assigned route, even up to this our time, our place.

But springing originally from the elements of humanity they are doomed sooner or later necessarily to meet again in her elements; springing from special wants, special necessities, and from peculiar frailties common to her nature, they can meet but in the general, the universal want, the philosophic element of humanity.

But it is time to leave the walks of general philosophy, to enter on the examination of those that are peculiar to the task assigned us: the philosophy, the theory, the truths of fever. It was by the Coan sage, we think, that the first elementary and the first imperishable truths were spoken, when he affirmed that fever was an effort of nature to expel some offending cause, or humor, from the body. Now this sentiment, so far as it goes, we hold in the abstract to be true; but the sage has failed in his explanations of its modus operandi; he was compelled to fail, to fall short of the full clearing up of the subject, for such a thing would have been without the pale of the circumstances of his existence, going ahead of the minutiæ of the sciences, the knowledge of which minutiæ is indispensable with the full, the clear, the transparent view of the theme.

His notions of the four elements, of blood, of phlegm, of yellow and of black bile, modern researches compel us to lay aside; while his leading, his elementary, his philosophic elements, will still stand. His views upon diet, exercise, and the influence of malaria in producing diseases, are for the most part based upon sound experience. Here he errs again when he dips into the minutiæ of explanation. From this doctrine of the four elementary humors have emanated the doctrines of Galen, and with varied modifications of all the humorists down to this day, receiving continually the lights of the minutiæ of science, as the sciences progressed.

But it would be trespassing on the time, the patience, and the good sense of the reader, to go into a detailed account of the varied grades and shades of light that belong to the different champions of the humoralists' schools: suffice it to say, that disease was by some laid at the feet of the elements of fire, by others of water, of phlegm, of acid, of bile, and of flatus, &c.

From the idea of flatus, with the Greeks, probably originated those numerous conjectures, phantoms, ideas, which at different times, different places, have assumed the various names of Spiritus, Anima, Neuma, Soul, Spirit Vita, Metis, Phanus, Eros, Cronus, Ulomus, Chusorus, Aura, Aroma, Vis Medicatrix Naturæ, et cetera. Now, under any or all of these titles do we recognize an element of truth, but that element has not yet been fully evolved. At this time, at this very hour while we write, is this phantom, this phenomenon in one of its protean forms, held up in wonder to the admiring gaze of the populace, by the followers of Mesmer. But we have not time to expatiate on this feature in the phenomena of the neumena of humanity.—That more properly belongs to our next series.

For the sake of brevity we have thought fit to link together some of the rival chains of thought. Let us then hold up to view the Rushites, the depletives, with the Brunonians, in modern nomenclature the Thompsonians, the steamers. Standing at the distance that we do, and beholding the movements of these rival captains, and their well armed followers, on the battle-field, recalls to our mind a passage from a poet of Rome, one of the favorites with us in the days of our boyhood, (dum stulti vitant alia vitia currunt in contraria,) while the one is running depletion to excess, the other is running on the opposite extreme, as though men could not perish as well by suffocation as by exhaustion—alias, as well by fire as by the sword.

"Veritas jacet inter extremas;" truth lies in the middle.

As to the Cookites, and the solidists, we see but little choice between them; to us both parties seem to have taken results in the depurative efforts of nature for their causes.

The one locates fever in the liver, and attempts to prove it by a very fanciful flourish about the portal circle in the circulation of the blood; while the other locates it in the mucous membrane of the stomach and intestines, and rests its proof on his numerous autopses. As to the results of their different modes of practice, again we see no choice. From our own personal observations on the theatre of life, we are led to believe that the one as many souls has purged away as the other bodies saved.

But a word to the enlightened founder of solidism.— When the immortal Broussais of Paris had reviewed the history of medicine, and with great skill, and with great judgment, criticised the labors and the theories of every predecessor, and upon their ruins based his localized views of fever, he then went on to demonstrate its truth by his numerous autopses; he thought, no doubt, that he had reached the terminus of thought; the bantling he christened (as par excellence) the physiological doctrine, and the world has accepted it under that specious title. But to us it only serves to recal to our mind a passage from the inspired author of our text, "The wisdom of man is folly, for he taketh the wise in their own craftiness."

The rigid mental discipline common in the schools of medicine throughout continental Europe, while they tend to perfection in the manipulations of art, either in surgery or medicine, are well calculated to circumscribe, to trammel, the native spontaneity of thought and general expanse of mind, so indispensably necessary for philosophic generalization, and progression in science. Thus we are enabled clearly to see the influence of the force of circumstances, which compelled Broussais to blunder. His physiology is based on anatomy; his pathology on his physiology, and his autopses served only to confirm him in error; he had not learned so to abstract himself from the purely physical man, as to see and to comprehend the laws of his neumena and phenomena, alias his vitality, or in other words again, he could not compass the whole man, in connexion with the whole series of causes and their consequences; therefore he took a result of fever for its cause.

What then is fever? We conceive it to be an effort of the conservative powers of nature, inherent in all animated creatures, to sustain its own integrity from the deleterious operations of causes, of whatever kind, by which it may be assailed; in this sense we make fever in its essence a unit; while in its phenomena, its physiognomy, it is multiform; and that multiformity of character proportioned to the peculiarity of constitutions, and circumstances of existence, and the nature of the varied causes or agents that are made to stamp diseased impressions on individual sensibility, or the sensibility of particular organs, particular tissues of his complicated machinery; which machinery should ever be considered as a unit, one whole, although composed of many parts, united by indissoluble laws of unity: the nervous chords, the true, the only medium of that much used, much abused, and illy comprehended term, called sympathy.

The difficulties, we should not say errors, in the labors of all who have preceded us, consisted, we conceive, in two reasons; the one is, that the elements of man, of medicine, and of nature, were not sufficiently evolved; the other in the want of development of mind, the ability, the liberty, the expanse of thought, to enable them at a single coup de œil, to compass the whole man, to comprehend the harmony of contrariety, to behold the unity of variety that dwells within him. Or, in other words, they have been like unto certain eastern reviewers, of certain philosophic thoughts on certain earthly phenomena, called cholera Asiatica, whose intellects being too limited, too local to comprehend a phenomenon which encompassed the whole earth, "very shrewdly suspected that in the same category should be included the whole of the balance of us." Now, since the reviewers have failed to comprehend our thoughts on a feature in the physiognomy of humanity, we have concluded again to try them with some thoughts on a single phenomenon in the physiognomy of man; or, using the words of the inspired author of our text, "Meats have we offered them, but find that to milk they must return."—Paul's Epist. to the Cor., chap. iii, verse 2d.

But it is time to leave the follies of the learned, and look to nature as the fount of light. Too long has man the world beguiled by promises of art; too few have looked to nature's walks, to see, to read the modest dame; the still, the secret and the silent ways, the sure, the lasting operations of her laws.

Through spectacles of books the world has looked from times beginning, down; it is time to lay aside the mask; let nature speak to nature now unmasked. But man, frail man, will say it is wrong to strip the damsel of her gown. We write for men; their voice we must obey. Then let the maiden stand not bare, but covered with a veil.

But to the labors of our task let us return once more, for on us now the duties fall to make our footing sure. We have wrought up man into one complete, one perfect whole, one living mass of organized machinery.

Now, inasmuch as this treatise is intended for general reading and extended usefulness, to go to the families and firesides of the community, the great body politic, more than the learned world, we conceive it to be our duty in the illustrations of our theme, in the applications of our theory to practice, the result of which is the only proper test of truth, to dip as little as possible into the mysteries of minutiæ—that is, into the play of atomic phenomena, atomic affinities—as such a course would serve only to embarrass the tender mind, and be productive of no real utility.

What, then, is health, but the harmonious play of all the solid structure, the equable and harmonious play of all the fluid matters, the healthy response of every surface, of every organ, to its natural, its healthy and its appropriate stimuli?

What, then, is disease, but an interruption of this play,

in some way, in any way, in every way, as the case may be?

Diseased action—that is, a departure from the healthy action—may result from many causes, and in very many ways. We shall, in the first place, enumerate the avenues of offending causes, and then proceed to mention some of them, merely for the purposes of illustration; for it would be going entirely beyond the spirit and intent of this treatise, to attempt a full and complete narration of causes, or of their modes of operating, as such a view would require the compass of many volumes. We shall therefore content ourselves with citing such only as are most familiar to the common reader, and such as are best calculated to give him a clearer view of the nature of disease, that he may the better see the indications of cure, and thus be enabled to vary his steps in the use of remedial agents, so as to bring about a return to healthy action, in the safest way, in the shortest space of time, and with the least possiple detriment to the constitutions of his patients.

The prime causes of all febrile diseases we conceive to operate on or to pass into the system through the following avenues, viz:

1st. Through the nostrils, the larynx, and the lungs.

2d. The whole extent of the cutaneous surface, that is, of the skin, whose offices, in many respects, are very analogous to that of the lungs; indeed, the inner surface of the lungs should be considered but as a continuation of the skin, in the light of a reflected membrane, so altered in structure as to perform an additional duty, viz: the medium of generating heat.

3d. The mouth, the pharynx, the stomach and intestines; and

4th. The senses,—commonly called the five senses,—that is to say, the sense of seeing, of smelling, of tasting, of hearing, and, lastly, of touch.

In the first place, let us take under consideration the liability to deranged action through the medium of the lungs, the breathing organs. Diseased action may be produced in the breathing organs themselves, from the mere extremes of temperature, or, what is more common, from the sudden transitions of temperature; or it may, again, result from the presence of gases positively deleterious to the organization, or from the absence of natural stimuli; those elements that constitute pure atmospheric air, so indispensably necessary to life and to health. When fevers result from any of the above-named causes, they are likely, under proper treatment, to be of short duration.

But there is still another way in which fever (commonly called essential fever) is produced; we mean those classes of fever produced by the absorption of malaria—that is, the imbibing the mephitic gases that emanate from the debris of vegetable and animal matter, or both combined. These fruitful sources of disease insinuate themselves into the animal organization, to make a marked impression on the whole man, without leaving any demonstrable traces in the particular structure through which they pass, or by which they are imbibed, viz: the skin and the lungs.

Now the system may be charged with the seeds of disease, that is, malaria, for weeks, yea, even for months, and still never be ripened into action; because it generally requires the operation of some exciting or proximate cause or causes, acting on the predisposed organization, to develope the disease: that is, to produce a departure from the natural, the regular, the healthy and sympathetic play of all the structure. The prime impression, then, is made on the brain—the centre, the fountain of all sentient phenomena. Indeed, but for cerebral and nervous sensibility, we should not be the subjects of disease at all.

It has been asserted, by Dr. Rush, that during the prevalence of epidemic bilious and yellow fevers, in the city of Philadelphia, that persons who were strongly charged or predisposed to fever, could readily discover it in the odor of their hands, by merely rubbing them together. We have frequently experienced the same thing ourselves.

But we should not overlook the disturbances of the depurative process, or functions of the lungs, as a source of fever. The deleterious effects of sudden transitions of temperature may so modify the lining of the internal reflected membrane of the lungs, as to impair its ability for receiving the oxygen of the atmosphere, and, at the same time, of transmitting the elements that should be thrown out through this waste way. Again, imperfect digestion disturbs the assimilation of the blood in the lungs, and in this way may prove a source of disease to the lungs, and consequently give rise to fever. But of this we shall speak more fully when we have under consideration the functions of the stomach and intestines.

It is, we believe, principally through the medium of the lungs, or breathing organs, that all those febrile diseases, called contagious diseases, are propagated; such as measles, small-pox, mumps, whooping-cough, and the like.

We come, next, to take under consideration the liability of the system to take on febrile diseases through the medium of the cutaneous surfaces—that is, the skin. The skin is well known, throughout its entire extent, to be an absorbing surface, under certain exigencies of the animal economy. For example, when the communication to the stomach, through the gullet, or œsophagus, is obstructed, and the individual is suffering much from thirst, then that want can be measurably supplied by sponging the surface of the body with water of suitable temperature, or by bathing. It is by virtue of this law that we are enabled to reconcile the fact, that poultry, sheep, hogs, and even cattle, can live for some time, and even fatten, too, when cut off from their regular and accustomed supplies of water to drink. They then take it from the atmosphere. From the foregoing facts are we led to the belief that malaria may, in like manner, be imbibed by the skin, and thus enter the circulation, whether such malaria be held in solution or in a state of suspension, merely, in water, or in atmospheric air.

But the most frequent, the most common, and the most demonstrable way, in which febrile action is induced through the interrupted functions of the skin, is the sudden transitions of temperature, particularly the impression of cold and humid atmospheres. These causes operate by putting a stop to both sensible and insensible perspiration, which we have already shown to be the most extensive, and as essential an outlet or waste-way for the redundant or useless matters of the system, as any excretory organ of the whole animal economy.

But, happily for man, the skin possesses within itself the power, in a most eminent degree, of adapting itself to the surrounding circumstances in which it is placed. There are, however, constitutional peculiarities in the textures and faculties of the cutaneous surfaces of different races of men. The African race, for example, have a more highly reticulated surface than the Caucasian, or other races of men; hence the stronger odor of the exhalations from their bodies, even under the same clime and the same mode of living. Hence, in all probability, their comparative immunity from the deleterious impressions of malaria; the depurative offices of their skin being more actively performed.

We come now to the consideration of the mouth, the stomach, and the intestines, as natural inlets of disease, particularly the seeds of febrile diseases; this we shall trace through the medium of the food. By this term we mean now to include all the necessary ingesta to sustain life, both solid and liquid, and aeriform fluids.

Food, although it be continually required to meet the exigencies of the system, may be and frequently is instrumental in the production of disease, in one or many of the following ways, viz.: first, by too long fasting, or the scantiness of nutritious matter in the food taken, or its indigestible form or nature; or, again, the want of the particular elements most needed at the time by the particular individual. The first impression of long fasting is the sense of hunger in the stomach, then of fulness and pain in the forehead, with a general sense of languor or debility; next the fever comes. Now, this fever is the result of the simple irritation of the brain from not having received its accustomed stimuli; the same results we have frequently witnessed from the stomach's not having received its accustomed kind of food; for example, milk in place of coffee for breakfast.

What now is best to be done? The doctor comes; bleed, puke, purge and sweat, or administer a mess of meats, soups, tea or coffee, as the accustomed habits say.

The food, the ingesta, the alimentaria may be productive of disease from mere excess of quantity, whether it be in a solid or liquid form. The over-distention simply may paralyze the action of the stomach. Again, when the ingesta is too much for the gastric secretions to save from the play of chemic laws; that is of natural decomposition, in other words, of indigestion, then the food becomes a source of disease; now, this result may take place in the stomach, or it may not be felt until the food reaches the intestines, then you may look out for colics and for bowel complaints, and lastly, for fevers. Such fevers would be strictly symptomatic; but of this we can say no more, as our business is to explain idiopathic or essential fevers.

The uses of the saliva and the objects to be accomplished by mastication, we think have been but imperfectly understood until now. The recent experiments of Professor Leibig have thrown much valuable new light on this subject. The learned professor asserts that the viscid nature of saliva is intended in the economy of nature to envelope globules of atmospheric air, and thus by masticating our food, we introduce quantities of oxygen into the stomach to pass from thence into the circulation to maintain the slow combustion so necessary for the production of animal heat. The professor further states that one main object in ruminating animals is to unite an additional quantity of oxygen with their food.

Now, if this be the fact, and we do not question it, the reader can readily conceive how it is that malaria, which is inseparably united with the atmosphere, finds its way with the food into the circulation.

Whoever has witnessed the ravages of what is called milk-sickness on cattle, horses, hogs, dogs, men, and even vultures, can readily conceive that poison may enter by the mouth and stomach into the whole organic mass.

We have witnessed its effects repeatedly, and on a pretty liberal scale, but of this we may speak hereafter.

It would be going beyond the intended limits of this treatise, to attempt to show the many elements and the many ways in which diseases or even febrile diseases may be induced through the medium of the extended catalogue of drinks and aliments; yet we will make one other remark before we leave this division of the subject. It is that a mere deficiency in the liquid elements in the system may prove a source of disease, as we have repeatedly witnessed when water was scarce, or was of such quality that it was only taken when pressed by very imperious calls of nature to allay thirst. Water is known to be continually required to maintain a proper fluidity in the blood. In warm weather particularly, and to laboring men, it is constantly expended by the exhalations from the skin and the lungs.

It is a fact well known to the profession, that when the serum, the fluid elements of the blood, had been wasted through the stomach, the bowels, and the skin, during the reign of the recent epidemic Asiatic cholera, that many individuals who had thus run into collapse, were again resuscitated, restored to life and to health, by merely injecting simple water or salt and water into their veins.

SENSES.

We come next and lastly to the consideration of the five senses, as avenues of disease. This investigation involves all mental emotions and phenomena, or, to speak more properly, all encephalic (brain) movements and perturbations, and the laws of sympathy thereunto belonging.

First, then, let us commence with the olfactories, the nose and the lining membrane thereof. While none but the natural sound and healthy emanations from fruits, from flowers, from men and animals floating in the atmosphere impinge on the organ of scent, all is well. Indeed, who is it that has not felt a pleasurable exaltation of brain, of thought, and through it of the whole organism from inhaling the odors of nature's laboratory, at the opening of the spring, or on a ramble over the spice islands of the south and east. Now, should we but change the scene, and let the olfactories meet, on every hill and every plain, in street, alley and the main, nought but mephitic gases of the dead, of men, of animals and plants, of whatever kind, of whatever hue, then the perturbation comes, the fever of the brain. Just so with the organ of vision: while the eye rests on pleasing scenes, then all is well. But when moral and physical putrefaction meets the eye wherever we turn, then comes the perturbation of the brain; delirium first and fever next succeeds, associations wild and horrid fill the whole machine, and onwards, onwards moves to death, from whence he came.

TASTE.

The direct and sympathetic associations of taste are either or both very frequent causes of mental perturbations, and even of physical convulsions, as we have frequently witnessed, and occasionally experienced ourselves.

Who is there that has never lost a meal from having swallowed, or even having imagined themselves to have swallowed, with their meats, milk, or other drinks, a fly or some more loathsome object? I recollect once in the days of my boyhood to have taken a few grains of calomel in a piece of preserved pear. Now this occurred while I labored under a gastritis, or inflammation of the stomach. More than thirty years have elapsed, and to this day my stomach would reject a pear, and, if the calomel were added, probably a gastritis would ensue.

We have heard a story of a learned medical professor, whose native modesty, in the juvenile period of his life, once compelled him, while at the festive board of a friend, to take down a chick from the egg, that had been cooked through mistake; and what is still more strange, (as the story goes,) it stuck. But we question much if that stomach has ever had a fondness for eggs, in any way, since.

HEARING.

The sense of hearing comes next in order, which is the last to die—that is, to leave us. This sense plays an important part in the drama of life. The deaf man is always serious—for the most part, melancholy; while the blind man plays the fiddle, whistles, sings, dances, and is talkative and gay. The immortal Homer, the blind poet of Greece, sang his Iliad, and Odyssey too, long after he had lost his sight Milton wrote his Paradise Lost after he had become blind.

The ear, then, as a medium of intelligence, is not less important than the eye. Through this channel may the passions, the emotions, the mental perturbations,—yea, all manner of physical and moral actions, either for good or for evil,—be produced. The tones of the orchestra, falling on the ears of the auditory, are made to elevate or depress, at the will of the performers. Just so the power of speech. The narrator, or orator, now inspires with hope, now gladdens with joy; anon, he fills with despair, or maddens into rage: then comes the fever of the combat, or the fever of disease.

TOUCH.

But there is still another sense which claims our especial regard. We mean the sense of touch, or the impressibility of man by the surrounding circumstances, or factitious causes. Man, in a state of nature and of nudity, is a very different animal from man dressed up and put in houses. The well-dressed, light-headed civilian hears of, or beholds, with astonishment, the debaucheries and excesses of the naked aboriginal, or debased African; the brutal Otaheitan, or the inhabitant of remote Polynesia. But not so with the philosopher: he comprehends the reasons for all these things, and wisely concludes, that

―"Whatever is, is right;"

that it is of necessity; and that you, Mr. Civilian, would

be astonished to find, with a change of circumstances, how soon you would learn to drink brandy, eat fish-blubber and horse-beef, and appreciate the delicacies of train-oil.

But it is time to come a little nearer home—to every-day experience. There are varied grades and shades of susceptibility and impressibility among ourselves; for example: the stings of venomous insects, or the handling of poisonous plants, do not affect us all alike; one man is proof against spiders, wasps, and bees, while another is laid up with fever by black gnats and mosquitoes. Some handle the poisonous oak (rus toxacadendron) with impunity, while others are laid up with eruptive fever by it: but none entirely resist the poison of the rattle-snake, the cotton-moth, or the mad dog.

"Now this is all a mystery; yet no mystery, too:
That which, to me, no mystery is, still mystery is to you."

Again, we observe very different susceptibilities and impressibilities in different individuals, and, indeed, in whole families, to contagious and infectious diseases; some taking on diseased action from the slightest contact, while others resist entirely. These facts we have known exemplified, in an eminent degree, in syphilis. But to offer explanations of these things, would be going beyond the limits of this work.

CHAPTER III.

In this chapter we shall endeavor to explain the author's views and opinions in regard to the common theories and practices heretofore adopted in the treatment of fevers; and endeavor to demonstrate the folly and irrationality of the varied modes of practice pursued under the influence of these theories. We shall commence with some comments on the depletive remedies. First. The use and abuse of the lancet. Second. The use and abuse of emetics. Third. The use and abuse of cathartics. Fourth. The use and abuse of diaphoretics: and conclude this chapter with some moral and intellectual views on the use of stimulants.

Having, in the preceding chapter, given a brief summary of the animal economy, and dwelt somewhat on the offices of those organs most involved in the phenomena of fever, we shall now attempt to prove, to the satisfaction of every unprejudiced mind, the error and impropriety of attempting to cure fevers, mainly, by depletion; that is, by bleeding, puking, purging, sweating—nauseating drugs, and the like.

It will not be denied by the followers of the anti-phlogistic schools, that they believe that fevers are almost all of a more or less inflammatory character; or that febrile existence, in their estimation, implies a state of exaltation of one or more of the organs of life: and that they consequently infer, from this view of the subject, that relief is to be sought for and obtained by and through the agency of remedies more or less depletive in their operations; that is to say, bleeding, puking, purging, sweating, nauseating remedies, and the like.

Now, while we are free to admit a state of irritation, a state of perturbation, and even more, a state of exaltation, for the time being, in one or more organs—one or more tissues, we shall endeavor to show, that it is not best to depend on depletive measures to restore the system to its lost salutary balance and healthy tonic action. For while we admit a perturbed, and even accelerated arterial action to exist in some of the organs, some of the tissues, during the paroxysms of fever, we contend that this accelerated local, or local and general *arterial action*, both combined, is the result of a loss of balance of the whole system, accompanied by a more or less enfeebled tone, and debilitated action of a part, or of the whole economy.

While we believe in the use of remedies, and give our assent to the salutary influence of remedial agents of the varied kinds that may have been heretofore brought into use, we would wish never to misunderstand or to run counter to the indications, the calls, the laws of nature, as unfolded in every individual case. We clearly comprehend, from our knowledge of the laws of supply and waste, in what way the followers of the depletive, the anti-phlogistic schools, have achieved the restoration of the lost balance, (the cessation of febrile disease;) but we contend that the depletive course, alone, is not the best, the safest, the surest, and the shortest way, to re-establish the normal action. So, also, we stand opposed to all those enthusiasts in the healing art who have been so rash as to think, and even to say, that we should take the case out of nature's hands into our own, and treat it according to the rules of art: for when the indications of cure are not strictly clear to the understanding, we then hold it safest and soundest to adopt the maxim of an aged medical friend, that "the error of omission is less culpable than that of commission." Then let us wait, and carefully observe until nature speaks out her own wants.

The depletists contend that their treatment is necessary and proper, if not to subdue inflammation, to guard against it; hence they take blood. The febrile heat and hurried action still continuing, they administer pukes, they say to expel morbific matter, and thereby subdue the disease. The heat of the skin and perturbed action still continuing, they administer purgatives, still to reduce the fever and to rid the system of morbific matters. The fever still runs on, they repeat their bleedings, emetics or cathartics, still to reduce or to eliminate morbific matters from the stomach, bowels, or gall-bladder, under the title of vitiated bile. But the fever still hangs on. They now begin to tighten the reins of government, and hold up a little; in the language of their grave consultations, these remedies they say have been pushed as far as the subject can possibly bear. Well, what next? Now comes either a course of nauseating and sweating drugs, or else the alterative doses of blue mass or calomel. By this time the race is nearly run; the patient either begins to mend in spite of the doctors, or retreats from their custody. Because there is evidently a hot and dry skin, thirst, often heat and burning sensation in the stomach and bowels, a quick, fretful, and irritated condition of the pulse, with more or less of pain, they contend that there is more or less of an inflammatory diathesis. As plausible as this argument may appear, it proves but little in support of the position taken, even in a theoretical point of view, as we shall attempt to show. In the first place, we hold that no fever proper is strictly of an active inflammatory character. Our proof is as follows:

All real and acknowledged inflammatory affections in the natural and unbiassed order of such phenomenon, run their course and come to a crisis in neither more nor less than eight or ten days. This law is so precise and notorious, that the ancients from their experience settled down on the ninth day, as the fixed period to arrive at a crisis. But when the old practitioners attempted to apply this law to fevers proper, they erred. Hence at this period of time the idea of critical days has nearly run out of use. Now, we still contend that this law holds good in acute pleurisies, fractures, and in all cases of fever from mechanic violence. The same law is manifested in the exanthemata, (eruptive diseases,) such as small-pox, measles, &c.

These diseases are known to all medical men to have a prescribed course to run, and the intelligent practitioner aims to conduct them to a salutary crisis.

But not so with fever proper. Yellow fever, plague, cold plague, typhoid fevers, and other forms of putrid fever, such as camp, jail, hospital fever, and the like, (to which might be added cholera morbus,) are all the natural and legitimate offspring of human folly, often kill their subjects in a day or two; while again they run ten, fifteen, or twenty days, or more, before the attending physicians can say whether the patients will recover or not. Milder grades of disease, such as common bilious, and mild typhus fevers, though they sometimes terminate life in a few days, not unfrequently run a month or six weeks before any one can say that they have even reached a crisis. Fevers then bear some analogy to ill-conditioned sores and ulcers having no fixed period for coming to a crisis. Fevers, however, are always of a general character, while these sores and ulcers may be either of a general or local nature, or both combined. But their continuance most probably depends on a debilitated and abnormal or irregular action in the depurative processes of the system; that is, in the play of the secretory and absorbent vessels.

The vital force being enfeebled, or the vital fluid (the blood) not containing the proper elements, or its elements not being in their natural and healthy ratio, the consequence will be inaction, that is, defective vital secretions; hence in such cases we rarely see a due proportion of animal heat, soreness, or inflammation in those parts; never the proper quantity and quality of well-digested pus (matter) and well-formed granulations until some favorable change is produced either by nature or by art; and this change is much more certainly and speedily made by such agents as will equalize the excitement, and purify the secretions, without debilitating the general system, than by bleeding, puking, and purging. When the ulcers or sores are of a local character, general treatment may not be necessary; but the applications should be alterative and deobstruent, astringents, tonics, or medicines more or less stimulant should be applied.

But it will be asked, if fever is not inflammatory what is its character?

We would say that fever is a disease of irritation; or, if you prefer it, and will allow the expression, we would go so far as to admit that it may be a disease of sub-acute inflammation. But fever never runs up into active inflammation. Secondly, although there is a hot, dry skin, thirst, often heat and burning sensations in the stomach and bowels, a quick, fretful, irritated condition of the pulse, with more or less pain; still we contend that there is not a general preternatural excitement in the system. On the contrary, that there is a general diminished action, and a general diminution of tone.

When the organs of supply, that is, the absorbent vessels, act with abnormal energy, that is, an energy too great for the organs of waste; that is, the organs of elimination and of exhalation, viz.: the skin, kidneys, and lungs; then the phenomenon of fevers takes place, that is, the circulation is perturbed, the skin becomes hot and dry, in other words, the equilibrium is disturbed, the healthy balance lost. Now, whenever this state of things occurs from the causes that produce fever proper, we contend that while the vital action is in excess, in the one class of vessels, it is in a proportionate torpor in the other class, and vice versa. So these oscillations continue to take place, constituting the remissions and paroxysms of fever, of diseased phenomena; until, by the unaided conservative powers of nature, or through the wisely directed agencies of art, the whole economy settles down to the natural equilibrium, the healthy balance again, or else terminates in death. Now these vessels, that is, the vessels of supply and waste, are in one sense antagonistical in their action; so that when the stomach and bowels are acted on by pukes and purges, the exhalants of the skin, lungs and kidneys too, are proportionally inactive or torpid.

Suppression of their accustomed functions takes place for want of the matter to eliminate, they having been thus directed to another channel; indeed the prime elements are wasted by this process—that is, the regular supply is for the time being cut off.

But it is further contended that thirst is a sign of inflammation. It was probably the existence of this symptom in the epidemic Asiatic cholera, which induced Broussais to administer cold drinks, and even ice, to his patients. To disprove this position, it will only be necessary to cite a few common occurrences familiar to the experience of almost every man, any one of which facts is worth more than a thousand theories. Whoever has suffered long in hot weather for want of water, as many travellers and soldiers have done, have found their skins hot, dry, and the sense of thirst insufferably great; so also, whoever has witnessed the war-worn soldier or the citizen weltering in his own blood, and dying from the loss of it, could not fail to observe the animal heat departing from his skin, with the failing of his pulse, while at the same time his cries for cold water became greater and greater to the last. Now, could any one be so stupid as to think or to say, in either of these situations, because the skin was hot and dry, or the thirst great, or both, or thirst with neither of the other conditions, that the sufferer was the subject of inflammation of any kind, or in any tissue? The thirst in either of these situations is demonstrably the consequence of a deficiency of the fluid elements of the blood.

Some as hot and dry skins as we have ever felt, were in low, protracted cases of fever, where there was evident debility, and much prostration in every part of the body. Every man familiar with fevers must have witnessed the same thing.

The hot and burning sensations occasionally experienced in the stomach and bowels, are often more distressing in the last than in the first stages of disease, when there is evidently general debility. It rarely happens in fever that the pulse is any other than a fretful and irritated one, increased in frequency to be sure—for a quick pulse is frequently indicative of a general debility—the circulation having to make up in speed what it wants in volume and in value. It may be full and soft, but is rarely if ever increased in force.

The pain ever attendant on fever is much more frequently the consequence of too little than of too much action in the general system. Witness the long train of painful nervous affections, acknowledged to be the offspring of an irritable condition of the nervous system, attended with more or less debility of the muscular fibres.

The neuralgia, for example, such as chronic rheumatisms, nervous colics, nervous sick headach, periodical headach or sun pain, tic douloureux, et cetera, all of which are of this class of disease; constituting a very considerable proportion of the pains that we suffer.

From what has been heretofore said, we feel a confident assurance, that the attentive reader will concur with us in saying, that to attempt to cure fevers proper, exclusively or mainly by bleeding, puking and purging, is irrational, unphilosophical, and at variance with acknowledged principles of human physiology.

Now, since it is admitted by all enlightened physiologists, that the skin, the kidneys, and the lungs, are the three great waste-ways for the redundant matters of the system, though there be several others of minor importance in point of amount or weight of matter eliminated, such as seminal secretions, and the matter of thought, the passions, &c.—that is, the imponderable fluids expended in thought and other encephelic (of the brain) phenomena;—we think that with these facts, these laws constantly in view, it will not be a difficult task to demonstrate the errors, heretofore committed by medical men, in the treatment of fevers, when they have relied mainly on bleeding, puking or purging, or a union of them all, to cure fevers.

While we admit the efficacy of all these classes of remedies, in certain cases, we wish to show the error of all those who have depended on them as remedies exclusively.

BLOOD-LETTING.

Let us commence with the use of the lancet;—whoever will bear in mind the physiological view of supply and of waste, can readily perceive that since the blood is both the medium of supply and of waste, it should be abstracted with great caution, and that we should never lose sight of the necessity of supplying it with new elements; that is, we should look to the proper supply of food, and of drink, and the necessary performance of the function of digestion in due time, to meet the demand of the economy that is to supply its waste.

The proper use of the lancet in all fevers proper, we conceive to be restricted to plethoric subjects: we mean persons of vascular plethora—and young subjects, whose recuperative powers will the better justify it;—in such subjects, when the victims of fever, our practice has been, and our settled convictions still are, that it is best to take off so much blood only as may be necessary to relieve the circulating system of abnormal tension; that is, to give to the circulating fluids their mature and accustomed free and easy play, and no more; and this should be done at as early a stage of the disease as its necessities may be pointed out. This opinion is the natural result of a combined experience of seventy-four years—that is to say, forty-six years for the one, and twenty-eight for the other.

EMETICS.

The indications for the use of emetics we hold to be two, and two only, viz: First, the evacuation of the contents of the stomach, either on account of its excessive fullness, or on account of the indigestible nature of its contents;—secondly, with a view to its revolutionizing and relaxing effects, whereby the waste-ways of the system are unlocked for a time, and the general economy is thus afforded an opportunity of resuming its lost healthy balance. Now, when fever is symptomatic, or even when it is in its proper character, and the causes, both prime and proximate, have been slight, or the constitutional stamina in the individual is very good, we have frequently found the diseased action cut short by the simple operation of a single emetic; when such result follows the use of an emetic, the patient needs no more. But when an emetic fails of the accomplishment of so desirable an end, we are opposed to its repetition, because it has achieved all the good that we had a right to expect from it, and the system is now prepared for the use of other remedies, more natural and far more efficient, as our experience has abundantly testified;—we mean that class of remedies called tonics and sodorifics. Whoever will bear in mind the operation of the natural law, that the waste-ways of morbific or redundant matters is through the lungs, the kidneys and the skin, and that the skin is the most considerable and important of the three, cannot fail to comprehend the propriety of these remarks; for so long as you irritate the stomach by emetic and nauseating drugs, just so long you suspend the action of the natural law of depuration; and so long, too, do you cut off the necessary supply of new elementary matters, which can only enter through the digestive process. In other words, he who repeats improperly, profligately sports with vital organization; and when this course is persisted in, as we to our mortification have been compelled occasionally to witness, under the direction of some of our intermeddling brethren, until the organic tissues were so much exhausted, and the stock of vital elements on hand had become too much reduced for the recuperative powers of life to reinstate itself, death becomes the inevitable consequence.

If any one should feel disposed to question the comparative utility of the two systems of practice, we have only to put to him the following question, and let his own experience answer it: Have you ever witnessed a genial and general perspiration coming over your patients, whether spontaneously or from the interference of art, and continuing for five or six hours, without a sensible mitigation of the symptoms—and that, too, without half the distress and the prostration that would have ensued from the same reduction of fever, (could it be achieved,) by the use of nauseating and puking agents?

We are well aware of the fact, that the suppression of the healthy depurations through their natural waste-ways, in fevers, not unfrequently, indeed very commonly, becomes a cause of local irritation to the stomach and bowels; the morbific or redundant matters seeking an exit through this channel, rather than through their natural outlets. In this way we can readily perceive how it is that that which, in the commencement of disease, is merely irritation, can, after a short continuance, become inflammation; constituting what Broussais and his followers call gastritis, or enteritis, or gastro enteritis, as the case may be: which occurrences they gravely lay down in their writings as the causes of fever. But we contend that the fever exists before the inflammation, and that it is always co-existent with the period of irritation.

If these views be correct, then how absurd must it not appear to increase the local irritation in the stomach and bowels by the repetition of emetics? It is not uncommon to see an attack of autumnal fever, of any kind, commence with a spontaneous and distressing vomiting. Now, could any one acquainted with the laws of healthy action, and, at the same time, with the laws of revulsion of the depurative functions, under such circumstances as have been just cited, think of administering tartar emetic, or active emetics of any kind? Would not common sense and reason instruct them to cast off the redundant matters from the stomach by the mere use of diluents, and then immediately set about to quiet its morbid irritation, and to throw the force of the circulation to the surface of the body as soon as possible, and thereby save the suffering organ from the danger of inflammation?

By gently moving the bowels, in any way, under such circumstances, you might diffuse the irritation over so extended a surface of the alimentary canal as to relieve any particular points or portions of it from the danger of great local distress. This course, which in many cases is necessary, and even the best step to be taken, is, at all times, preferable to relying on the repetition of emetics, or even nauseating drugs.

There is still another idea in febrile diseases, which has long haunted the minds of practitioners and the people; that is, the quantity and quality of the bile. Having but some vague notions of diseased secretions of the liver,—which have been expressed by the terms vitiated and redundant bile,—they imagine that the patient should be puked or purged so long as the liver continued its morbid secretions, or that some bad consequence must inevitably follow. The thought seems not to have occurred to them, that the secretions are partly kept up by the use of their medicines, as well as by the continuance of the disease; and that there are other means of relieving the patient besides those of puking and purging. But of this we shall speak more fully under the next head.

We might be charged with having too little regard for public opinion, if, while on this point of our subject, we should pass unnoticed the practice of the steamers—the Thompsonians. The followers of Thompson place great reliance on the virtues of the lobelia inflata. With this article of the materia medica we have, long since, had some acquaintance, and more or less of personal intimacy. Besides its emetic properties, it possesses, more or less, the properties of a sialogue. In its effects and its operations it bears a striking analogy to tobacco. We think, from what we have witnessed of its effects, that it is much better adapted to the treatment of croups and catarrhal affections, than to febrile diseases. As an emetic, in fever we should give a preference to ipecacuanha.

CATHARTICS.

Purgatives, in all ages and in all countries, have been justly enrolled on the list of important remedial agents, and in the hands of different practitioners, the different articles of this class of remedies have obtained a varied celebrity. While some have preferred individual articles, in their simple, uncombined state, others have exerted their ingenuity to find the best articles, and to make the best possible combinations of them. Hence has resulted the long catalogues of patent purgatives, and anti-bilious pills, whose miraculous virtues have filled our papers with certificates of their infallible cures; from the celebrated Lee's anti-bilious, down to Cook's R. A. C.'s. We find one sect of doctors deriding the use of the mineral cathartics, while another sect are extolling them as the Sampsons of the materia medica: some contending, exclusively, for the offspring of the vegetable kingdom, and asserting that all things else are poisonous to the animal economy, (such are the botanic doctors,—one would think that such men had not exactly kept pace with the progress of organic chemistry;)—some there are, again, who give a decided preference to the saline cathartics. So we find one class of practitioners (the Hamiltonians and the Cookites, for example,) promising the greatest possible good, in the treatment of fevers, from the use of purgatives alone; while many of the French medical writers scarcely admit their efficacy at all. In this labyrinth of doubt, who shall dare assert, "I am the light, I am the way."

In a word, mankind have projected almost as many ways to health as to heaven; while, in truth, there is but the one way to either.

If we were permitted to give our opinion on the use of cathartics in febrile diseases, we would dwell less upon the particular article than upon its dose and its repetition. Almost any article of the class may by suitable combinations be made to set easy on the stomach, and to operate gently on the bowels; yet every individual stomach, especially if it has often been under the care of *Doctors*, has its aversions, (we could not say its partialities,) and these circumstances we think always worthy of attention. In our choice, then, we should be in a great measure guided by the antipathies of the patient, and the circumstances and symptoms at the time being; sometimes the mercurials should be preferred, sometimes the vegetable, at other times salines, and not unfrequently a combination would be preferable, according to the particular modified action desired to be produced in the case.

With our settled physiological and pathological views, we have but little use for cathartics at all; and when used, we would desire to have them operate efficiently, but as mildly (that is, giving as little local irritation) as possible. To us the indications for their use would seem to be, first, where there was constipation of the bowels, or fulness of the alimentary canal, then evacuate; secondly, when the irritation of fever was spending its force mainly on the brain, then we should use cathartics, with a view not merely to evacuate and to diffuse the irritation over a larger surface of the system, but to produce revulsions from the brain to the alimentary canal, and thus prepare the patient for the better operation of other remedies.

We are not ignorant of the fact that fevers have been repeatedly cured by the mere repetition of cathartics, for we have had the same thing occur occasionally under our own experience; we know, that with good constitutions, the work of depuration and the ultimate restoration of the equilibrium, may be achieved through the medium of the stomach, bowels and liver.

But to accomplish this much time must be consumed, great suffering endured, and considerable emaciation and consequent prostration of physical tone produced; and when the constitutional stamina of individuals is defective, death is not unfrequently the result of such a circuitous route to health.

But the depletists, especially the purging sectarians, contend that there is great acrimony, vitiation, and redundancy of bilious matter in the system, that can be eliminated only by purging.

We will not deny that the secretions in fever are generally abnormal; but we do contend, that the departure from the healthy action as frequently consists in a defective as in a redundant secretion. We are even willing to admit that the bile formed under the febrile action is not often strictly healthy in its properties; but the admission of this fact does not lead us to infer, with the many who have expressed their opinions, that the acrid bile is the cause of the fever; we conceive that to be as clearly a consequence, as is the inflammation of the mucous membrane of the stomach and bowels, so much relied on as a proof of the soundness of their doctrines, by the lovers of the autopsic mode of settling the laws of vital phenomena.

Much has been said of the necessity of discharging morbific matters; and the liver has been much more censured for the part it plays in febrile diseases than it really deserves.

The mass of mankind have been almost urged to the belief, that the existence of bile was inimical to health; and if to it should be added the qualifying expression, vitiated, from the lips of grave medical philosophers, then it becomes truly alarming.

Now, while we admit that the liver in the discharge of its functional duties frequently departs during fevers from its healthy labors, and that sick stomach, head-ach and vomiting are sometimes occasioned from this cause, yet, we know that a regular and plentiful supply of bile is as necessary for the process of digestion and a healthy existence as any other named secretion for its destined office: nor is it more liable to vitiation or decay than other secretions.

It is known in its natural envelope, the gall-bladder, or in an inspissated state, under favorable circumstances, to be preserved for any length of time; indeed, it has long been in use as a vulgar and popular remedy for colics, dyspepsias, and fever; and we have such faith in the efficacy of sound healthy bile, as to believe that it will, ere long, find favor even with the learned.

The occurrence of high-colored urine, and the yellow tinge of the skin, so common in bilious fevers, jaundice, and yellow fever, should not be ascribed so much to the superabundance of the secretions of the liver as to the inverted or retrograde action of the absorbents. The bile in these cases we conceive to pass directly from the liver and the gall-bladder back into the circulation, instead of first entering the alimentary canal, and then passing through the absorbents and lacteals, whose mouths are spread out on the surfaces of the stomach and intestines.

The unpleasant symptoms attendant in these conditions of the system, we are disposed to ascribe more to the loss of balance in the great functions of organic life, and the enfeebled energies of the brain and nervous system, than to the mere presence of misplaced secretions—for bile misplaced is no more than any other secretion or element;— and the only reason why it has attracted so much attention, we conceive to be because of its color, it being the only one of the numerous secretions which in becoming misplaced is rendered visible to the eye.

Every body is familiar with the retrograde action of the lacteals and absorbents in cholera morbus, and more especially in Asiatic cholera, where the lacteals and absorbents were not only employed in emptying their own contents, but through them the blood-vessels themselves were exhausted of their serum, their fluid elements, to be thrown off by the stomach and the bowels.

Now, having witnessed these facts, and comprehending

as we do the operation of the natural laws of health, we object to treating fevers mainly by cathartics and emetics, first, because such a course would be inverting nature's laws, and secondly, because we have found a much better and safer way to arrive at the same desired result—namely, the use of tonics and sudorifics.

But that sect of partisans known to the public under the imposing title of mercurial doctors, will contend that they have and can achieve more good by the judicious use of mercurials, than any one can do with tonics and sudorifics, such men often deceive themselves and the public too, from vague notions connected with the color and consistency of the stools. Those who have observed them closely in the routine of their professional toils, have found them administering calomel for almost all purposes; for example, if the operations are thin, they give calomel, if otherwise, they give calomel still; if white, calomel; if dark, calomel; if green, calomel; if yellow, calomel still;* in a word, they seem to have the same blind attachment to calomel that certain topers have to whiskey; it is their toy for joy, their remedy for grief;

"For hot or cold, wet or dry,
There's nought so good as oil of rye."

To us the color and consistence of the evacuations serve to throw some light, not only on the condition of the organs themselves involved, but on the state of perturbation of the general system likewise. The color of the evacuations is more or less modified by the operations of three causes, viz.: the food we eat, the nature of the secretions for the time being, and the chemical character of the drugs taken. Some articles of food, in conjunction with the remedies taken, will cause pale or even white discharges, others green, some a yellowish cast, while others again dark, brown, or black, and each may still be equally healthy.

---

* Many valuable lives, we have no doubt, have been sacrificed to the erroneous ideas attached to dark discharges; such appearances being as much the effect of the calomel as of the nature of the disease.

While we admit the virtues of calomel and blue mass, we would wish to limit the abuse of them. The calomel doctors who have made the liver the focus of all fevers, and calomel the panacea, while they contemn the idea of a catholicon in medicine, still continue to apply mercury in some shape or other, in some dose or other, in every stage and every form of fever. It is their cathartic, their alterative, their salivant, their solvent, and even their tonic.

There is one disease, and one only, which we have not been able to treat satisfactorily without it; we mean lues venerea, or French pox. Over this disease it seems to exercise some specific virtues; but even in this disease we have been accustomed to use it very guardedly.

The great facility with which doctors are fabricated now-a-days, and the innumerable swarms that are turned out annually from the many factories now scattered over the whole surface of the civilized globe; is one of the many reasons that have induced us thus to place in the hands of the people the result of our researches and experience, that they may be the better enabled to understand the laws of self-preservation, and may the better appreciate the comparative value of the labors of their medical advisers.

But we have not yet taken leave of the mercurialists. The extent to which calomel and blue mass have been administered during the last twenty-five or thirty years, is so great, and the ratio that has been mal-administered so enormous, that it is high time for humanity to raise her voice, either to disarm her heroes of the weapons of death, or to withdraw her subjects from the field. In what part of this vast continent can any man cast his eyes, and not behold the grave of some victim of its pestilential powers? Where can a social club convene, that does not contain some living monument of its wrath?

It is, indeed, the most insidious of all known poisons. The poison tree of Java, the serpent, the arsenic and the prussic acids, either give timely warnings of their presence, or destroy their victims at once. But not so with the god Mercury or his knights: those who listen with credulity to their whispers of fancy, or pursue with alacrity their phantoms of hope, are doomed sooner or later to awaken in the realities of despair; for when once the victim of their remorseless grasp, neither prayers, tears, time, nor antidotes will ever remove the spell; for every rain that falls, every wind that blows, will ever tell through all their aching bones.

To such of our readers as have dived deep into that department of the arcana of nature called laws of propagation, we may safely assert, that mercurial disease is not solely confined to the individual sufferers; but its effects are, in a greater or less degree, revived in their offspring. Every body knows that like begets like, yet all do not know that this law holds good even to the particular condition of body or mind, (we had like to have said brain,) at the particular moment of vivification. But these things we must leave to posterity to settle.

DIAPHORETICS.

We come next to treat of that class of remedies whose action on the animal economy is in strict unison with nature's laws. In casting over in our minds the great ruling and controlling powers of organic life, we discover two very important movements in vital phenomena.

The one we shall call the centripetal, the other the centrifugal; the one a concentration of the energies of the vital forces to the internal surfaces of relation; the other, the conducting of the same forces to the external surfaces, (or what might be more strictly speaking, to the periphery of vital action,) there to eliminate or to bid adieu to all those elements which, having served the purposes of life, are no longer needed, and whose continuance, indeed, would be oppressive to the system. In the right knowledge and the right exercise of a controlling power over these phenomena of vital action, consists all the secrets of health and of disease.

Sudorifics and diaphoretics are those medicines which, being taken internally, increase the sensible and insensible exhalations from the skin. This effect may be produced in any one of many ways, or more certainly by a combination of means; to exemplify, external heat alone may produce this effect; the use of diluents, the use of stimulants proper, (we mean not irritants, see chapter on medicines,) the use of the vegetable, mineral, and alkaline diaphoretics proper; and the many combinations that may be made of them. Of this numerous class of remedial agents, the discoveries now in progress in organic chemistry, will lead us to make the most judicious choice. Our past experience has led us to give a decided preference to the vegetable and alkaline, or a union of the two. This class of remedies, when rightly understood, comprises two other classes of human ordination, viz.: expectorants and diuretics, for collectively these agents are used for the same purpose, namely, to unlock and to maintain the equable action of the three great waste-ways, the lungs, kidneys, and skin; that is to say, in the natural order, they are but different members of the same family; hence under one set of circumstances diaphoretics are made to act diuretically, and vice versa; under another set of circumstances, diuretics act as diaphoretics.

To explain more fully: Squill, digitalis, the alkaline salts of potash, soda, and ammonia, any one, or a combination of these articles,—in conjunction with warm diluents, such as flax-seed, or other simple herb teas,—with a warm atmosphere, a warmly clad skin, or tepid bathing, either general or partial, will cause an increased exhalation or discharge from the skin. But use the same articles, and change the circumstances to a cold skin, cold extremities,—a passive condition, or a condition of passive exercise, such as a ride of a cold day,—and substitute malt liquors. Give cider, or even the free use of weak wines, and you may expect an increased diuresis. Again, if you place a patient in a medium situation as regards the protection and temperature of the body, and use the same articles in such combinations as will cause the nauseating drugs to make a sensible impression, you may expect to have the greater burthen of the offices of depuration thrown upon the lungs, that is, you will have the expectorant effect.

In certain healthy conditions and natural exigencies of the body, simple cold water is the most prompt and salutary sudorific known; for example: In hot weather, under circumstances of great labor and fatigue, when cut off from regular supplies of water until the skin becomes hot, feverish and dry, and the sense of suffering from thirst excessively great, a pint or more of good, pure, cool water promptly allays all sense of distress; and its administration is promptly followed by a general flow of perspirable matter from every pore of the whole surface of the body. In the case just cited, the experience of the world goes to prove that the remedy is not only prompt, but even pleasurable; just so should be the operation of all remedial agents in the treatment of fevers, under the guidance of wisdom. But the folly of man, and the madness of medicine, have ever caused him to be too local, too circumscribed, too bounded, and too much inflated with a partial discovery of isolated truths, to seek the harmony of all the truths which belong even to a single series in the phenomena of nature. Hence, when Brown had discovered an element of truth in the use of stimulants, he ran his theory, this element of truth, to excess, and, fortunately for the world, he fell an early victim to his own partial discovery.

From the ashes of a Brown have arisen the theories of a Jennings and a Thompson, and other members of the same family, to play a more rational part, and to approach some nearer to the temple of truth, on a modified and an extended scale: Hence the application of stimulants, both externally and internally, by drugs and by fire; and these, too, aided by their distressing and depressing, yet efficient ally, the far-famed lobelia. The errors of the steamers, to us, seem to consist, first, in their not being able to discover the particular cases to which their routine was best adapted, and their indiscriminate application of their remedies to all manner of cases; secondly, in the excess to which their remedies have been used. When, in their faint glimpses of the laws of life, they had learned how to make an impression on the skin, and observed the salutary results which, occasionally, followed therefrom, they immediately presumed too much; and were led to take up the erroneous idea, that, by forcing the living actions through the instrumentality of pepper, brandy, myrrh, and external heat, to achieve whatever they desired by the mere force of arms. Like unto some simple men, (in every country to be found,) relying on the length and strength of their purses to make wise men, or gentlemen of their sons, by the mere power of wealth! As though the God of Nature could be bribed to vary his eternal laws, to please the gatherers of gold.

Now while we admit the essential differences that belong to stimulants, tonics, and diaphoretics, we, at the same time, contend that they all act in unison with nature's laws, and that, under proper restrictions and right circumstances, they constitute our chief reliance for restoring the lost balance to the circulation, and the play of healthy action to all the functions of organic life. When rightly used, they all tend to excite and to sustain the healthy, concatenated chain of action in the whole system, and to direct the energies of the vital forces to the surface of the body; that is, to facilitate the action of the natural and healthful depurations, which being rightly maintained, will in due time relieve the system of deranged, irritated febrile action.

From an attentive view of the foregoing explanations, in connection with what we have already said in our chapter on the laws of the animal economy, we are led to the belief that the intelligent reader cannot fail to comprehend the comparative value of the several modes that have been resorted to for the cure of febrile diseases. All those who have relied on bleeding, puking or purging, by using, repeatedly, any one of them, or resorting to the whole of those means, conjointly, have practised an unnecessary waste of the elements of life, and not that alone: but by the improper repetition of emetics or cathartics, they have inverted the natural action of the system;—thus producing a retrograde action of the lacteals and absorbents, which inverted action, in connection with the local irritation made on the mucous membranes of the stomach and bowels, by their use, we conceive to be the real causes of the congestion and inflammation, so commonly to be found on post-mortem examinations.

Before we take leave of this subject, it would be well to make some remarks on the controlling powers of the moral agencies on the secretions. To all who have been attentive observers of human phenomena, the fact must be notorious, that the impressions of fear not only increase the urinary secretions, but, not unfrequently, result in untimely evacuations from the bladder and the bowels. Such spectacles have we repeatedly witnessed, in by-gone days, under the uplifted rod of the school-master, or the dog-whip of the sportsman. These phenomena are always attended with more or less of a temporary chill, contraction, and consequent suppression of the exhalations from the skin, whereby the fluids are thrown more abundantly on the kidneys.

But when this same impression is protracted and carried to the highest pitch, then are we called to witness an inverted action of the lacteals and absorbents, which are promptly followed by copious and rapid evacuations from the stomach and bowels. But of this we shall speak more fully under the head of cholera.

We can conceive of but two general causes of disease; that is febrile proper, and one, a particular condition of the system, the other, a peculiar state of the atmosphere, and it is to the modifying influence of these causes, separately and conjointly, that we are to look for the shades and grades of fever.

Many are the volumes that have been already written on the subject of malaria, and the other predisposing causes of disease, yet still has this subtle element eluded our grasp; of its intrinsic essence we know but little; of its modus operandi on the animal economy, we are likewise in the dark; with its sources, that is, the felicitous circumstances for generating deleterious gases, have we formed some acquaintance, and with its effects on the human frame have we all had some, more or less, of personal intimacy. It may be, that to know the prime sources of disease, and to understand its effects, is all that is necessary and proper that we should know; however, we flatter ourselves that chemical and philosophical researches will not cease to be made, until all of these mysteries are cleared up to our view.

One thing certain is, that every breath we breathe, every step we take, and every evolution of the mind, is a more or less predisposing or exciting cause to either healthy or unhealthy action in the system. Nor do we often know, with absolute certainty, whether they are to be for the better or the worse. It is from the lessons of wisdom and experience alone, that we can learn how best to deport ourselves. Health, whether of body or mind, (and it takes the two to make the whole man,) are much more closely allied, more inseparably linked together, than the mass of mankind have ever yet thought. Either or both, under the guidance of reason, will find the greatest share of health and of happiness in pursuing a just medium in all things. He who shuts himself up in a house, from fear of the influence of the sun, the wind, &c., is at least as subject to disease, as he who regularly and fearlessly faces them all; or he that does not take bodily exercise or lives on too spare and meagre a diet, from a fear of wearing himself out, or under the vain hope of prolonging his existence, is about as likely to cut short the thread of life, as he who obeys the instinctive impulses of his animal desires.

STIMULANTS.

Sudorifics, tonics, and stimulants, are all centrifugal in their effects, all having a tendency to facilitate and sustain the circulation of the blood, to excite and to maintain the natural secretions and exhalations from the body; and not that alone, but to counteract the enfeebled, the irritated, the irregular and the spasmodic actions attendant on fevers. Of sudorifics we have already spoken; of tonics we shall speak more fully in our next chapter; but of stimulants we must have something to say before we close the present. The present state of knowledge as conveyed in the classification of remedies, and the use of terms, renders it necessary for us to explain what we mean by the expression stimulants proper. The word stimulus, or stimulant, has by most writers been indiscriminately applied to whatever would excite the living tissue. In this sense emetics, cathartics, cantharides, &c., are all stimulants. But we shall confine the use of the term to those articles only, which excite or exalt the system in a manner only congenial to its own healthy laws; all other excitants we shall consider as irritants.

When we look to the origin, the history of stimulants proper, we find them springing only from those elements that are capable of sustaining animal life; and the quality of the stimulus always modified by the quality of the elements from which it is obtained, and the chemical aptitude and skill with which it is elaborated. The grades of nutriment, of permanency, and of diffusibility of stimuli, is the result of the formative powers of the processes of fermentation and distillation, and the elements used. Thus we obtain wine, cider, malt-liquors, rum, brandy, whiskey, and their subdivisions.

But the weakness of man, in his approximation to truth, has ever kept him vacillating from one extreme to another, from the extreme of confidence to that of distrust, from confident hope to unnecessary fear. When the process of distillation was first successfully put in use, some of the philosophers of that day verily believed that they had discovered the secret of human immortality. So fascinating, indeed, are its effects, that it readily found favour in every land. Now, since the distilled liquors have travelled the earth over, been tasted, tried, used and abused by all nations; now, while we write, are societies organized, and public speakers invited to proclaim to their fellow-men, the dangerous, the deleterious, and the deadly influence of intoxicating drinks; the drinks themselves calumniated, and held up to public view as man's vilest enemy; and are societies formed ready and willing to expunge from the list of valuable discoveries, and important goods of nature's bounties, the name, the laws of distillation. Thus verifying the words of Horace, "dum stulti vetant alia vitia current in contraria."

Whenever man shall acquire wisdom and virtue rightly to see, and rightly to appreciate, his own ignorance, and his own folly, then, and not till then, will he cease to abuse the munificence of Deity.

The very reasons for which the civilized world is now toiling to put down the use of stimulants, viz.: its excessive use, its abuse, is to us the strongest possible proof of its salubrity, of its efficacy; for if its elements, its action on the living atoms, had not been congenial to the laws of his nature, man would never have learned to have loved it so. But our opponents may say that all this is habit. If so, will they be so kind as to tell us why their patients and the world, have not yet in like manner contracted a fondness for calomel, tartar emetic, ipecac., or any other of the numerous drugs we call irritants? Malt liqnors, wine, cider, contain, in addition to their stimulant properties (their alchoholic elements) some nutritious matter; and even the alcohol itself, we have reason to believe, is consumed in the living actions; no portions of it having yet been detected in the excrements, the secretions, or exhalations from the body. By the aid of the light of chemical philosophy, are we now enabled to solve the fact that has been so frequently pronounced, that it is a slow poison.

A thorough knowledge of its modus operandi in the healthy economy has enabled us to comprehend in what way it operates beneficially in the diseased condition. When the vital forces are much enfeebled by disease, and the stock of alimentary matter necessary for the support of life and animal heat is much diminished, then the prudent use of stimuli operates beneficially, by allaying irritation, directing the vital forces to the capillaries; thereby restoring the lost equilibrium, while at the same time, it either nourishes the system, or at least prevents that waste of the animal matter that would otherwise result for the necessary maintenance of animal heat.

We hope that no one will infer from what we have said of the use or the modus operandi of stimulants, in the diseased condition, that we are advocates for its use as a luxury; far from it; we use it not ourselves, nor have we ever advocated its use in others. The result of our experience furthermore is, that however grateful, and however beneficial it may be to the enfeebled, the diseased, and the convalescent from fever; that they invariably lose their appetite for it with the return of strength and of health.

We would have its consumption strictly confined to remedial purposes. We are well aware of the fact that many unfortunate individuals have an ungovernable propensity for its use, even in their best health. This state of things we can readily trace to two sets of prime causes; the one, the organization of the brain; and the other, the circumstance of education: both of which could be easily remedied by the united efforts of philanthropy and wisdom.

CHAPTER IV.

THE AUTHOR'S PRACTICE AND TREATMENT IN THE CURE OF FEVERS.

HAVING stated in the preceding chapters our objections to all the various systems, doctrines, and modes of practice, that have been heretofore pursued, and dwelt at some length on some of the particular errors introduced into practice by our predecessors, such as the errors in bloodletting, puking, purging, &c., in the varied degrees and modes in which these measures have been applied to the treatment of fevers, we will now endeavor to unfold to the reader a very different, and as we honestly believe, a far better plan of treating fever of all types, from whatever causes they may spring, and under whatever forms they may appear: for to us, since we have learned to view man as a unit, all general diseases seem but a unit—so, consequently to us, fever is a unit.

Now, let us look back for a moment to what we have already said of health and of disease. Health is but the harmonious play of all the solid structure—the equable and harmonious play of all the fluid matters, the natural response of every surface, of every organ, to its natural, its healthy and its appropriate stimuli. What then is disease, but an interruption of this play, in some way, in any way, or in every way, as the case may be?

What, then, is fever? We conceive it to be an effort of the conservative powers of nature, inherent in all animated creatures, to sustain its own integrity from the deleterious operation of causes of whatever kind, by which it may be assailed. In this sense we make fever, in its essence, a unit, while in its phenomena, its physiognomy, it is multiform, and that multiformity of character proportionate to the peculiarity of constitutions and circumstances of existence and the nature of the varied causes or agents that are made to stamp a diseased impression on individual sensibility, or the sensibility of particular organs, particular tissues, of his complicated machinery: which machinery should ever be considered as a unit, one whole, although composed of many parts, united by indissoluble laws of unity, the nervous chords, the true, the only medium of that much used, much abused, and illy comprehended term, called sympathy.

Now, if the reader is capable of comprehending what has been already said, and will hold the truths already unfolded to his view ever present in his mind, he will find no difficulty in understanding and giving his assent to that which is to follow.

The phenomenon of fever you will recollect we have said is the result of general debility, attended with a loss of balance in the functions of supply and waste. This state of things impresses on the individual sensibility of the individual sufferer the assemblage of phenomena called fever, such as lassitude, heat, thirst, pain, restlessness, with a more or less perturbed and interrupted performance of all the functions of life, vegetative, animal and intellectual; in a word, a diseased or abnormal manifestation of some or all the functions of organic life. For centuries past have the industry and ingenuity of man been fruitlessly essayed to find the shortest, the safest and surest way to remedy this state of things. Born and reared as we have been under this state of collision of thought, and doomed by our calling to act as collaborators in the cause of science and of truth, we now find ourselves compelled by the lights both of experience and research, to feel confirmed in the propriety of discarding the theories of every predecessor, and with them their practices also;—because in our investigation of the laws of organic life, we think that we have discovered some modifying or remedial agents, capable of making more prompt, more specific, and more salutary impressions on the diseased subject, than any of the numerous measures heretofore relied on for the accomplishment of the same end.

These agents are called the vegetable alkaloids. To this family belong quinine, cinchonine, morphia—a class of remedies occupying the middle ground between that of the depletive and the (strictly speaking) stimulating remedies.

Upon the timely and judicious use of this class of remedies do we chiefly rely for the cure of all fevers; not denying ourselves, however, the benefit of any or all other remedies that science or experience may have pointed out as salutary and proper. Thus you see, that we have admitted the propriety of blood-letting in certain cases and under certain restrictions; so also have we admitted and recommended the use of emetics and cathartics, under particular circumstances and with suitable restrictions.— (See the respective heads in chapter 3d.)

But our main auxiliaries to the use of quinine are the vegetable and alkaline diaphoretics, and in cases of extreme prostration the use of stimulants, with the use of tonics. In all cases of local congestions, irritations and inflammations, we have both practised and advocated the propriety of topical bleeding by cups or by leeches—also the use of sinapisms and blisters: still, however, holding on to the regular use of tonics, with such auxiliaries as might be indicated in the particular case or state of the patient.

The pills which the author has prepared for sale for

several years past, and distributed under the name of "Sappington's Anti-Fever Pills," and which have deservedly acquired a character for efficacy in the cure of fevers, far surpassing that of any other article ever offered to the public, or any other plan of treatment before adopted, were simply composed of one grain of quinine each, three-fourths of a grain of liquorice, and one-fourth grain of myrrh, to which was added just so much of the oil of sassafras as would give to them an agreeable odor. The liquorice and myrrh were cheap and convenient articles of which to make the mass; they were not intended as articles of medicine at all, nor could they have had any sensible effect; the whole virtue of the pills consisted in the quinine alone. The medium dose directed in his prescriptions being uniformly one grain of quinine to an adult, and in that proportion for children, no unpleasant effects have ever within our knowledge resulted from mistakes being made in the use of the remedy, although they have been placed in the hands of persons of all descriptions, and recommended and used in all stages and in every form of fever to be met with in the limits of these United States—particularly those States lying in the great valley of the Mississippi, for the space of eight or ten years.

Although the author has vended pills to a large amount, and realized considerable sums of money by his sales, the people have also saved a great many dollars by using them; been relieved of much pain and suffering, and very many lives have no doubt been saved and prolonged. The author consideres himself driven to this alternative, more from motives of benevolence than from those of self-interest.

Knowing, as he did, the prejudices that existed against the medicine, he also knew that, had he published his opinions to the world in any other way than as he has done, and is now doing, that neither the public nor himself would have benefited much, if any, by it. But, from the manner that has been adopted, the full benefit is now given to the world; together with a great deal of other useful matter, that could not well have found a place in a newspaper, or common hand-bill.

The obstacles, with our predecessors and cotemporaries, to the discovery and adoption of what we hold to be truths, (that is, the aptitude of quinine to the cure of fever,) are two-fold; namely, a belief in the inflammatory nature of fever, in the first place, and, secondly, of a stimulating or inflammatory property in the nature of quinine. The error of their notions in regard to fever, we hope, has already been satisfactorily proven to the understanding of every intelligent reader; and it now only remains for us to show the fallacy of the other imaginary obstacles, and then the whole mystery may be considered as dispelled.

We know of but two ways by which we can settle, or put to the test of our senses,—that is, of our understanding,—the properties of bodies, of material things: The one is, the inferences to be drawn from their sensible impressions on living matter; the other is, the chemical manifestations displayed in relation to, or in conjunction with, the other things and circumstances.

Suppose, now, we submit the article of quinine to these tribunals, and see what will be the result of our examinations? Let us first hold it up in a chemical point of view.

What is quinine? It is the salt of the bark of a tree indigenous to the elevated lands of Peru, in South America. It is obtained by the processes of maceration, desiccation, and crystallization. It is not, then, a product of either fermentation or of distillation; it is not volatile: it is a fixed salt, not liable to waste by evaporation.

From whence are stimulants proper derived? They are all, either directly or indirectly, the offspring of nature, through the vegetative process; and are elaborated, purified and concentrated by human contrivances, under the natural laws of fermentation and of distillation. Hence comes camphor, porter, ale, cider, wine, rum, brandy, whiskey—the essential oils of all scented plants; to which might be added, ammonia, all stimulating articles, and all volatile and more or less perishable by evaporation. In the chemical view of the subject, then, we are led to infer, from the processes of obtaining, and from the facts of its comparative exemption from change under common atmospheric influences, that it does not possess those qualities common to the list of articles universally recognized as stimulants.

But there is still another way by which to arrive at truth: it is, the testimony of the facts of human experience, or of human observation on human sensibility; alias, the phenomena in living human matter.

Now, when we consult the pages of history, from the period of the first discovery of the virtues of the Peruvian bark, A. D., 1500, we find febrifuge properties ascribed to it. From that period to the present, in the hands of different chemists and different practitioners, have its properties, and its varied remedial uses, been differently represented. Still we find that the sum of the testimony—the sum of the experiments and researches, up to this day, have tended rather to advance, than to detract from its virtues; nearly all writers admitting its antiseptic and its tonic properties, while some in a limited sense were willing to ascribe to it febrifuge and alterative virtues. The weight of our own personal experience will go to show, and to give to it, all the virtues for which it has, as yet, obtained credit, and even more. In our hands, for years past, in some form or other, has it succeeded, in a far more eminent degree than any other article of the whole materia medica, in contending successfully with fever, of whatever type, and in whatever stage it has come before us. It would be trespassing both on the patience and the good sense of the candid reader, to attempt to lay before him any thing like a detailed account of our personal experience. But, for the satisfaction of those who are pleased with the reports of cases, we have thought fit to cite the following:

When we were attending medical lectures, in the city of Philadelphia, during the winter of 1814 and '15, there was a man in the hospital laboring under an attack of simple ague and fever, the paroxysms returning each day. This patient had been there at least three weeks; had no other disease; and, when the chill and fever were off, was able to get up and go about. This case had been treated, all the time, with common remedies; that is, with occasional pukes and purges, and with what we call refrigerating mixtures, during the fever, such as a solution of salts of tartar, or cream of tartar, with nauseating doses of emetic tartar, or ipecacuanha; and, in the entire absence of both chill and fever, with small, but seldom repeated, doses of the bark, from a fear of aggravating the fever, and, at the approach of each chill, a few drops of laudanum were given. I do not recollect distinctly, but think it probable that the lancet had been used occasionally, also. The bark and laudanum were gradually increased as the disease continued, but not sufficiently to make a sensible impression on the system, so as to obtain an ascendancy over the disease, as should always be done in the treatment of ague and fever. The hospital physician at the time, one of the professors of the University,—Dr. R. S. Barton,—invited me, one evening, to take tea with him. In the course of our conversation, he learned that I had been practising medicine for several years. He then mentioned to me the difficulty and uncertainty of the cure of ague and fever, in general, and named this case in particular. I was much pleased when he brought it up, and, with some reserve, stated, that if I had his patient in Tennessee, (where I then lived,) that I thought I could cure him in forty-eight hours, at furthest. He looked at me with some degree of astonishment:

"Then, pray," said he, "if it is not a secret, how would you treat the case?"

I advised the use of the bark and wine shortly after the sweating stage commenced, and to use as much of the bark as the stomach could bear, until a short time before the chill was expected to return, and then to increase the dose of laudanum or opium at least two or three-fold. The professor made "the experiment," (as he called it:) His patient had no return of either fever or chill. He was cured immediately.

It should be recollected that at that time quinine was not known.

Some time during the summer of 1840 I was called to see a Miss N., whose life was said to be despaired of. I found her the subject of a typhoid fever of ten or twelve days' standing. She was much emaciated, very feeble, and suffering with great restlessness, with occasional fits of delirium, her tongue dry, skin hot and dry, thirst great. I learned that there were two physicians in attendance: they had been and were then giving at stated intervals blue mass. I remarked to the mother of the lady that I could not wait to see the gentlemen in attendance in consultation; but that she might say to them, that I did not approve their course of treatment; that I would discontinue the use of the mercury; and put her immediately on the use of tonics and diaphoretics. If they thought fit, they could adopt that course; if not, and she thought fit to adopt it, that I would send her the medicine and prescription, and she might treat the case herself. Furthermore, that I was of opinion that if they persisted in the course they were on, she would lose her daughter; but that if she would put in execution my prescription, we should have her mending in a few days. What passed between the good lady and the doctors is of but little importance to the reader; suffice it to say, that I was promptly applied to for medicine and prescription.

I simply directed a grain of quinine to be given every two or three hours, and a solution of the alkaline mixtures of the supercarbonates of potash and soda in such quantities as would allay the patient's thirst. A few hours' use of these remedies excited a genial perspiration, with a return of healthy secretions to the tongue and fauces. I learned that by the next morning all sign of fever had fled, the patient commenced and continued to convalesce until her health was entirely restored. She has continued in the enjoyment of good health ever since up to this period. Were there any motive or any utility in it, we could go on to fill thousands of pages with reports of similar cases.

We have already asserted the belief that the salt of Peruvian bark was the best tonic, the best antiseptic, the best febrifuge, alterative and deobstruent with which we were acquainted, and that in our hands, in conjunction with suitable auxiliaries to meet particular indications, we had achieved more good in the treatment of fever, than with any other named article of the whole materia medica. We have expressed an opinion also adverse to the belief of its possessing strictly stimulating properties: its efficacy, we contend, resides purely in its tonic property; in other words, in its aptitude to the sustenance of the brain and the nervous system; which, in truth, is the primum mobile of all vital phenomena.*

Whoever would desire a more extended view and a better understanding of this part of our subject, should consult the lights of organic chemistry, particularly the recent labors of Professor Leibig.

Before we take leave of the general view of the subject, it would be well to adduce still another argument in support of the correctness of the general principles contended for. The argument is this: If the followers of the strictly depletive doctrines, the Rushites and Cookites, have done much good, succeeded well in the treatment of fevers, and if also their antipodes, the Brunonians, the Thompsonians, &c., have achieved half the wonders that they claim, occupying as we do the middle ground, the JUSTE MILLIEU, is it not reasonable to infer that we who accept the lights of both extremes and of all extremes, but who tenaciously hold on for the middle course, may be entitled to a modicum of the laurels won; to be placed at the feet of tonics and diaphoretics in the temples of Esculapius?

We are not only satisfied as to the curative powers of quinine, but we are disposed to ascribe to it preventive virtues also. To this conclusion are we led not only from experiments made in the author's own family; but from facts occurring in the experience of his travelling agents.

He has had for the last eight or ten years from fifteen

---

* Or it is possible that it may neutralize the virus of fever.

to twenty-five agents employed in the distribution of his pills, each travelling from three to six months every year. These agents have been sent to all those states and to such portions of them too, as were considered the most sickly; they were generally sent off early in the spring, and seldom returned earlier than June, July, or August, and not unfrequently set out again in the heat of summer to the most sickly regions of country. These agents were all instructed to use the pills occasionally as a means of protection against the influence of malaria, and there has never yet occurred a single instance in which any one of them has contracted a fever of any kind.

From these facts we are led to infer that if quinine was judiciously used in sickly countries and in sickly seasons, that such a thing as fevers of any type, would rarely if ever occur, excepting under circumstances of the combined operation of the many causes.

When quinine is used as a preventive, an adult should take a dose of one grain three or four times a day, until he takes twenty-five or thirty grains. This quantity should be taken every two, three, or four weeks, until the sickly season is over, or the epidemic has subsided. Children should take less in proportion to their age.

CHAPTER V.

THE AUTHOR'S VIEWS ON THE SUBJECT OF THE UNITY OF FEVERS.

WE have already expressed the opinion that fever was a unit, and assigned some general reasons for such a belief. But we shall, in this chapter, enter more fully into the details of the argument, and endeavor to show that all fevers are of one family, from the mildest form of intermittent, or ague and fever, down to the lowest grade, and most malignant type, of yellow fever—putrid fever; congestive, nervous, typhus, or whatever nomenclature you may please to adopt. We view all fevers as one continued chain of diseased phenomena, and the varied symptoms or modifications, as only so many different links, produced by some peculiar conditions of the atmosphere, or states of the system. Now, both of these modifying causes are incessantly changing, and from these changes originate all the apparent dissimilarity in the features of disease, while in its essential character it is ever the same; and every variety of it should be treated pretty much alike—that is, with the same classes of remedies, varying them only to suit the peculiarities of cases, and the grades of diseased manifestations.

We speak, here, of diseased manifestations, when left unbiassed, under the controlling agencies of natural causes. Very many of the worst features assumed in fever, are the result of mal-practices or hyper-medication. In all such cases, we have ever been of opinion that the patients would have fared much better in the hands of dame nature and the nurse, than under the officiousness of uninformed and intermeddling doctors. But the immortal Broussais, of Paris, has said, that there is one disease, at least, in which any practice is better than no practice, (Asiatic cholera.) About this we may speak hereafter.

As a proof of the unity of disease in fever, and that the reader may more fully satisfy himself of that fact, we will here give a summary of the most common and important symptoms in all fevers, which will show, most conclusively, that the symptoms of all fevers are the same, differing only in degrees of intensity, and that they are in proportion to the mildness or severity of the causes, and the peculiarities and the impressibilities of the constitutions in which they are manifested. There are, generally, several days of indisposition previous to the attack of all fevers. This is called the premonitory state. This state is known by loss of appetite, lassitude, a general restlessness, or sometimes an unusual drowsiness; more or less disturbed sleep; with a disinclination to action of any kind.

In the attack, in the onset of fevers, it rarely happens but that there are more or less of chilly sensations, attended with flushes of heat. Sometimes, these chilly feelings run into agues, or shakes; but with the advance of disease, or as the fever rises, the chilly sensations subside.

In the commencement of all fevers, it rarely happens that there is not more or less of aching pains over the whole body; predominating, however, in particular portions, such as the head, back, and limbs. Sometimes this pain is exquisitely distressing; but it is apt to moderate as the disease progresses, or as—in the language of the schools—the reaction becomes established.

In the onset of all fevers, there is more or less of lassitude, weakness, or sense of weariness: in some instances it is considerable; and this weakness continues to increase as the diseased action advances.

In the onset of all fevers, there is more or less of increased thirst; sometimes it is intensely great. This symptom also continues as an attendant on all fevers, but it is apt to moderate as the disease progresses. Although the tongue, lips, and even fauces, or throat, may become more dry in such cases, the desire for drink springs more from the unpleasant sensations of dryness, or suspended secretions in the structure just named, than from the actual cravings of the stomach; since patients in this situation take only a swallow or two at a time, while in some other conditions no amount that could be retained by the stomach would satisfy the desire.

In the onset of all fevers, there is more or less loss of appetite for food; sometimes an aversion to food, amounting to nausea, or sick stomach, without vomiting, at other times with vomiting, and occasionally attended with both puking and purging: and it is well known that there is little or no appetite for food during the progress of fever.

In the first and earlier stages of all fevers, except in the lowest grade of cold plague, yellow, putrid, or typhus fever, and even sometimes in these, the pulse is apt to be not only quicker than natural, but irritated and fretful; giving, oftentimes, the delusive appearance of increased force, when, in reality, the force is diminished, and the circulation, in such cases, labors to make up in frequency, or speed, what it wants in force. But as the disease advances, and the patient becomes weaker, the pulse becomes still quicker, weaker, and smaller, making but very feeble resistance to the pressure of the fingers, and evincing clearly a want of force.

In the first stage of all fevers, the tongue becomes covered with a whitish coat, or fur. This, however, is not always discoverable in the onset of the disease, but becomes observable in the course of a few days; and if the fever is not checked, but suffered to run into another stage, then the tongue is apt to assume a yellowish brown appearance. But should the fever be of a lower grade, or more malignant character,—particularly should it partake of the putrid form, such as yellow fever, putrid fever, or the like, —then the tongue is apt to assume a dark brown or black color. The casting off these different colored coats from the tongue should ever be considered as a favorable omen. In the last stages of all fevers, the tongue, teeth, and lips are apt to become exceedingly dry, and oftentimes encrusted with a dark, sticky, gummy matter. In some more rare cases, the tongue assumes a different appearance from any of those that have been mentioned; that is, it assumes a smooth, glossy, red appearance. This is apt to take place after many days' continuance of fevers, or about the last stages of disease, or after relapses. Whenever this state of the tongue occurs, we have generally found the cases to be more tedious and more dangerous.

In some cases of fever, there is a roaring sound, or tingling, in the ears. This is most common in typhus or nervous fevers, but it does, occasionally, occur in any form of fever.

Delirium is a common and a very distressing symptom in all fevers. This particular symptom is more the offspring of peculiar organization, than the nature of external causes: some individuals, and some whole families, being prone to delirium under fever, from whatsoever causes or under whatever type; while other individuals are capable of passing through any form of fever without much, or any, very appreciable derangement of the functions of the organs of thought.

In the first stages of all fevers there is apt to be a kind or grade of disturbance of mind, not amounting to delirium, that is, a slumbering or dozing condition, that the patient is more conscious of than his attendants. This symptom, indicating but a slight departure from the normal state, is of but little consequence.

But as the disease progresses in its stages and grades of prostration, the delirium assumes a different and more distressing character; the observing attendants now discover a considerable derangement in the faculties of the brain, of which the patient himself is not conscious. He frequently lies to some extent in a state of stupefaction, often hard of hearing, so much so that it is difficult to arouse him, and when aroused to make yourself comprehended by him; indifferent to the exterior world, he makes you short responses, and drops into his slumbers again. In more advanced stages you find him picking at his fingers, and at the bed-clothes, sometimes entirely stripping himself of all covering; again, we hear him uttering incoherent words and manifesting a desire to be up and going about, when he is not even able to stand on his feet. In such patients we are apt to witness a creeping or twitching of the muscles of the arms and legs, (what is called sub sultus tendinum, by the doctors,) the voice becomes weak, and sometimes unnatural, with a wild, vacant expression of the countenance.

There is still another form of delirium, which also occasionally attends the last stages of fevers, and indicates a more dangerous condition than the one just mentioned; this is attended with incessant watching, the patient's sleep leaves him, his hearing becomes even more acute than natural, he is startled at every sound, and has imaginary and for the most part distressing images continually passing before his eyes. In all other particulars his condition is pretty much the same as in the state just before mentioned.

Now, as the delirium and muscular agitations or twitchings increase in proportion to the duration of the disease and the physical prostration of the patients, these results must be ascribed to the general exhaustion and consequent debility of the whole physical organization, and not to an increased action of the brain, the heart, the blood-vessels, or any other part of the body, as a large portion of the medical faculty would have you to believe.

In fevers, generally, we observe some more or less sense of heat in the stomach and bowels; we observe, also, an increased color and more scanty secretion of urine.

In the last stages of all fevers we occasionally witness involuntary discharges by stool and by urine; and in all forms of fever these are alike unfavorable symptoms, though not necessarily fatal, as individuals have recovered after such discharges from all manner of fevers.

In all fevers the salutary changes, that is, the crisis, is usually announced by the occurrence of very much the same phenomena; that is, nearly all the cases yield under a return of the salutary action of the depurative functions, particularly that of the skin.

Although the circulation of the blood has been long understood, and the indications to be drawn from the action of the pulse long studied, and many grave, lengthy, and learned discourses been delivered from the pulpits of the schools, yet still are the discrepancies of opinion upon this subject as great, even at this day, as at any former period of time. Such, too, must necessarily be the case, for two important reasons—the first is, that the faculty have not yet agreed even in the abstract, as to what constitutes the propriety or impropriety of taking blood; the second is, the difficulty which the mass of practitioners find in comprehending the influence of physical and moral causes on the phenomena of circulation in their patients. For want of a clear knowledge of all these things, do the most experienced and observant practitioners sometimes make blunders.

In the examinations of all cases with a view to the indications of cure, we should never fail to take into consideration all the symptoms of the case, as well as all the circumstances of causation. Among the many signs which lead us to a knowledge of the condition of the sick, there are none more uniformly important than those of the tongue and the skin; the strictest attention should therefore be paid to their state and condition.

As a proof that physicians know less about fever than is generally supposed, and less even than they themselves imagine, we hear them continually disputing about the names of fevers, of a country, a place, or a season, such as typhoid, congestive, and bilious fever—just as though they were all distinct diseases, and to be cured by widely varied remedies. The truth is, that the similarity of the symptoms in the early stages of all fevers is so strikingly great, that it is not a matter of astonishment that they should so often dispute about their classification. Many practitioners prescribe more from the appellation which they shall give to the assemblage of symptoms, than from a knowledge of what is taking place in the economy of their patients; they as often or oftener form their opinions as to the name or nature of a fever, from the season of the year in which it occurs, than from the symptoms which attend on it. We have known the fever of small-pox mistaken for that of malignant fever—the fever of measles treated for bilious fever. It is not, then, a matter of surprise to us, to find them mistaking one shade of autumnal fever for another, nor would such mistakes be a matter of much importance, provided they understood the nature of the fever in the general.

We are accustomed to see fevers assume the character called bilious, in warm seasons and in warm countries, while typhoid fevers are more common in the colder seasons and in the colder countries.

We have thought that fever was like unto man, its prototype, never stationary, always either in a state of progression or of retrocession, often varying much in its progress, but never fundamentally changing; often running regularly through the different grades of the particular type it may assume, but now and then running from one type to another—from a higher to a lower, or from a lower to a higher; that is, from the simple intermitting form to bilious or even typhus at one time, while at another time, from typhus to bilious, and finally ending in chills and fevers. Such things are not unfrequent occurrences in cases of relapses.

Notwithstanding our conviction as to the truth of the position, that there is a natural chain of connexion which binds all fevers together, yet still do we find it convenient for the purpose of making ourselves the easier and better understood by the reader, to adopt the common classification of fevers. Hence, in the succeeding chapters, we shall treat of the several varieties; commencing with the mildest forms of what is called summer and intermittent fevers, and ending with the lowest grades of fever, called cold plague or spotted fevers.

The objects in view in the course of this chapter have been mainly to show, by a brief summary of the general symptoms attendant on all fevers, the unity of disease, and in a general sense the identity of all fevers proper; and if in this attempt we have either failed or erred, fevers are still living and impartial witnesses, and will speak for themselves.

CHAPTER VI.

OF INTERMITTENT, OR AGUE AND FEVER.

We believe it is now universally admitted, that low, marshy lands, and all those countries or situations where the surface of the earth is such as to retain the waters that fall on it, either by virtue of its depression, its evenness of surface, or by the impervious nature of its clay, or where the waters of creeks and rivers are stagnated either by artificial or natural obstructions, are ever fruitful sources of that condition of atmosphere which generates in the human subject the types of fever called intermitting and remitting fevers.

As we are engaged in writing solely with a view to practical utility, we would consider it an unnecessary waste of the reader's time, here to enter into any investigation of the laws of malaria, the laws of vegetable and animal decomposition, or the theories of the agency of water and caloric in dissolving, elevating, and disseminating the ultimate elements of either salutary or deleterious matter.

The term intermittent, or ague and fever, is applied to that form of fever which is characterized by distinct and perfect intermissions, or periods of exemption from febrile symptoms. Having never yet been able to discover any utility in that extravagant love of words and of mere verbal displays, which has induced the nosologists to affix a name, a term, or a title, to every symptom, whether trivial or otherwise, that might perchance accompany this form of fever, we shall content ourselves with the introduction of those only that are the most common results of its natural periodicity; such as quotidian, tertian, quartan, and their subdivisions into double, treble: and so forth, and this division even, so far as the treatment is concerned, we consider of no importance, since in whatever form it may appear, its nature is the same, and the proper treatment, with but slight modifications, should ever be the same also.

We consider all fevers as intermittent in character, which effectually cool off between each paroxysm, whether preceded by chill or not, or where the chill and fever rise together, sometimes a paroxysm of fever of this kind continues not more than an hour or two, returning after a lapse of about twenty-four hours; at other times, the paroxysms are of much longer duration, lasting twenty-four or forty-eight hours without an intermission; and again, sometimes running on for three or four days; but whenever a paroxysm continues for two or three days, and then goes off entirely, it is not so apt to return.

The most common form of intermittent, however, is to have a chill or shake every day, or every other day, or every third or fourth, and followed by a fever of from two to ten or twelve hours' duration. A large portion of the fevers in these United States, partake more or less of the intermittent character, particularly in the southern and western states.

SYMPTOMS.

The symptoms of ague and fever are very similar to those of other forms of fever in the onset of the disease.

There are generally several days of predisposition or premonitory indications previous to the attack, unless in cases of relapse.

The attack usually commences with a sense of lassitude and weakness, with a yawning and stretching; quickly followed by coldness, rigors, and trembling; then comes a paleness and lividity of the extremities; laborious respiration, anxiety, nausea, sometimes vomiting; pulse frequent, small, and feeble, though sometimes more slow; thirst great; the skin generally sensibly corrugated, and of a more or less livid hue, urine pale and scanty. These symptoms constitute the first or cold stage; which often continuing for a longer or shorter time, is succeeded by a heat or redness of the skin, particularly of the face; the respiration becomes fuller, stronger, and more free; anxiety less, pulse fuller and stronger; thirst still great, with more or less pain of head, back, and the limbs. This stage is again succeeded by the third or sweating stage, when a remission of all the symptoms takes place under a more or less abundant perspiration, sometimes attended with an increased discharge of urine and dejections from the bowels.

The intermittent is justly considered the mildest form of fever, and when rightly treated in the commencement or before it has continued many days, is usually the most manageable form of fever that we have to contend with: but when neglected and suffered to run its course for a time, a long list of formidable diseases or results is apt to follow in its train, such as engorgements and enlargements of the spleen, pancreas, and liver; attended with febricula, indigestion, and not unfrequently followed by watery effusions or dropsies of the abdomen and of the whole body.

The intermittent form of fever occupies a much wider range than the medical faculty or the populace have as yet been aware of. To this type of disease do we trace the many anomalous cases of periodical pains in various parts of the body, attended with more or less of febrile symptoms, such as sun-pain, and very many muscular and neuralgic (nervous) affections of the limbs and other parts of the body.

TREATMENT.

Bleeding: This remedy has at no period in the history of medicine found many advocates in the treatment of intermittents, yet it has occasionally found favor with particular individuals, (Dr. Rush, for example, reports favorably of its use,) and we are not sure but that there are even at this time some individual practitioners who are partial to the use of this remedy. We can conceive of but a very few cases or situations in which it would be admissible and proper. Those cases are when the disease occurs in young and plethoric individuals, and in such subjects as have a constitutional proneness to particular congestions or inflammations; such as a disposition to apoplexy or congestion of the lungs. In such cases we have thought it would be a safe and proper practice to abstract just so much blood and no more, as to take off the excess of tension in the vascular system, which could be certainly done by one or two small bleedings, and then proceed to treat the case with the proper doses of tonics and diaphoretics.

EMETICS AND CATHARTICS.

For these classes of remedies, too, we can find but little use in the treatment of intermittents. Should spontaneous vomiting occur, then we can see no necessity for the administration of an emetic, for the stomach empties itself; and when there is neither sick stomach nor vomiting, we are still unable to see any good reason for producing such symptoms. But whenever a paroxysm of fever occurs on a stomach overloaded with food, and a puking ensues therefrom, then it is best to suffer the organ to empty itself before we attempt to compose it.

As to the use of cathartics, we are well aware that some of the learned professors of the schools have strongly advocated, and placed great reliance on them, under a belief that the disease was caused by a congestion in the liver, and that the use of drastic cathartics constituted the most efficient means of relieving that viscus: But we hope that we have already succeeded in convincing the reader of the fallacy of such reasoning. The principal inducement with us, in prescribing the use of an aperient or cathartic, would be, to relieve the patient of constipation, should such a state of things exist; for we believe that, under the proper treatment, the stomach and bowels should be left or kept as nearly in the normal, or healthy condition, as possible. Hence, in cases of looseness of bowels, we should use small doses of laudanum or paregoric; say, six, eight, or ten drops of laudanum, every six or eight hours, until checked, or an equivalent of paregoric: but if there is sick stomach, or vomiting, then use essence of peppermint, or some other cordial.

What, then, do we conceive necessary to be done?—that is the question. Simply to combat the fever by the use of tonics, aided with sudorific drinks, during the hot, or febrile stage, and prevent its recurrence by the continuance of the tonic remedies (quinine) during the intermission. For this purpose we have found one grain of quinine every two hours,—both day and night,—regularly administered through all stages,* sufficient for all salutary purposes; and if the dose were augmented to two grains, during the same period of time, we should apprehend no bad consequences therefrom. We have aided its action on the skin, during the hot stage, by the use of warm diaphoretic teas, such as sage, and Virginia snake-root, to which might be added a little red pepper, or sometimes

---

* The author has never failed, with this course, to relieve his patients in the course of two or three days.

the alkaline salts. So soon as a general perspiration is excited, or the febrile symptoms are caused to abate, then discontinue the use of the sudorifics, and continue that of the tonics alone.*

In all chronic diseases of the abdominal viscera, whether of the spleen, the pancreas, the liver, or dropsical effusions, arising either from neglect or mal-practices, whether attended with febricula (what is called inward fevers) or not, our practice has been, to use either the vegetable tonics or the tonic preparations of iron, in medium doses, two or three times a day, with occasional doses of blue mass or calomel; say, one or two grains once or twice per week. The same practice should be pursued in the treatment of similar chronic affections, arising out of any other fevers. [See chapter XVI.]

We have been more than surprised at the very liberal, not to say extravagant uses, that some of our brethren have recommended, and even made, of the sulphate of quinine. We learn, from the medical journals, that the sulphate of quinine has been administered, in from fifty to one hundred grain doses, with a view to remove obstructions of the spleen, &c., for the cure of intermittents. We consider this a wanton abuse of one of the best remedial agents known to the profession. We are at a loss to conceive on what grounds such doses can be justified, in any kind of cases. It reminds us of the enormous doses of blue mass, and of calomel, that were administered in many cases, and in many parts of these United States, during the prevalence of the Asiatic cholera. Dr. Eberle speaks of 4320 grains of calomel being given, in twenty-four hours, to one patient, and recommended it to be repeated in the next twenty-four hours, in a case of cholera. [See Eberle's Practice, page 558.]

In a letter from Dr. Lewis to Professor Mitchell, of

---

* As in this form of fever the patient is more liable to relapse than in any other, when once the disease is arrested, he would do well to take two or three doses of quinine a day, until his strength and complexion are restored.

Philadelphia, dated Paris, March, 1841, the following interesting statement is made:

"At the hospital of De La Pitie, I have seen the sulphate of quinine used in a wholesale manner for the treatment of intermittent fevers, supposed to be caused and dependent on the enlargement of the spleen. The doctrine is held that the fever cannot exist without the enlargement and derangement of this viscus.

"This theory has many disciples, and many enemies. To relieve this state of things, doses of fifty or one hundred grains of quinine are given, and with obvious effect. I have often very satisfactorily percussed the spleen, and marked its limits, before the administration of the medicine in the above doses, and, in twenty minutes after its administration, I have seen this organ very perceivably reduced in its whole circumference, and the paroxysms arrested or palliated in an incredibly short time."

The lessons of wisdom to be drawn from such a practice, go to establish three very important points: First, the safety and salubrity of quinine; secondly, a deobstruent quality in that drug; thirdly, that such is the wise and happy construction of the animal economy, that life is not necessarily the forfeit of mal-practice. The immunity from injury in such cases, we would attempt to account for, on the supposition that the whole force of the drug could not at once be brought into action on the living structure; and in this, the most favorable view that we can take of the subject, it would seem (to say the least of it) a want of economy in the use of the medicine.

CHAPTER VII.

OF COMMON BILIOUS OR BILIOUS REMITTENT FEVER.

From what has been already said of the unity of fever, in chapter 4th, the reader's mind must be prepared to receive the assertion, now sustained by all truly enlightened practitioners, that all fevers are more or less liable to run into one another, according to the influences of external causes, and the susceptibilities and impressibilities of individual subjects; that is, that observation has taught us the fact, that intermittents, remittents, inflammatory, bilious, congestive, typhus, and malignant yellow fevers, have all, in many instances, run into each other; so also have we seen, in the same locality and at the same time, the same season, different individuals the subjects of all the diversities of forms: for example, one patient has intermittent, another remittent, a third congestive, a fourth typhus, and so on with the endless subdivisions which belong to those generally comprehended terms.

From these remarks it will be readily inferred, that fevers are almost infinite in the varieties of shades and grades which they assume.

It is through the instrumentality of these truths that the world has been kept so long in the dark, by the wonderful fascinations of mystery, (the magic of words;) while fever has ever been a unit, one and the same phenomenon from the days of Hippocrates, or even of Adam, down to the present time; with, in truth, but slight appreciable changes or shades of difference, to correspond with the developements of humanity, man has created for it as many names, titles and dresses, as would fill the wardrobe of a modern city dandy.

The doctors and dandies have both been ever laboring to the maximum of their wits, but with this marked difference in the moving spirit of their toils—the one has ever been laboring to discover the truth, while the other is laboring to discover the best mode to conceal it.

Now, this state of things has originated from the limited and bounded nature of the human mind, which has ever compelled him first to toil, to develope, and to propagate isolated elements of truth, as a step preparatory to the ultimate explanation of the whole; since the harmony of these elements can only be seen by him who comprehends each and every individual atom or element of truth.

We come now to the consideration of that part of our theme which we have thought fit to call the second link in the general chain of fever, viz.: summer or autumnal fever. There have been about as many names given to this link in the chain as there have been modes of practice prescribed for its cure.

It has been called bilious, remitting bilious, intermitting bilious, inflammatory bilious, malignant bilious, &c. Of late years we have seen it crowned with a new title, the congestive fever, or the congestive bilious, or congestive intermittent, as though it were a new disease—the term congestive used as a discriminating symptom, as though it did not belong to all other fevers—for we cannot conceive of any fever without more or less congestion somewhere; the only difference then that we can perceive is, that this particular feature is more marked, more prominent than usual, for the disease all the time is the same old acquaintance we recollect oftentimes to have met with on the lowlands of Maryland and old Virginia, in the days of our boyhood. The doctors then called it malignant intermittent.

This form of fever is most prevalent in the marshy situations of warm countries, and in the warmer summer and autumnal seasons of all countries. Like other fevers it is usually preceded by more or less of premonitory symptoms, such as are common to other fevers. The attack is usually announced by chilly sensations, more or less distinct, and of a longer or shorter duration, sometimes amounting to an ague; these symptoms are succeeded by the ordinary symptoms of hurried respiration, pulse fretful and quick, for the most part full and soft; pain of the head, back and limbs, a general restlessness, nausea, and sometimes a vomiting of bilious matter; this is sometimes quite an obstinate and distressing symptom; the skin now becomes hot and dry, the thirst considerable, the patient usually desiring to drink more than the stomach can bear. These symptoms remit or abate once in every twenty-four hours, sometimes twice, but never go entirely off before a fresh attack ensues, so that the patient is never without some degree of fever; the remissions usually occur during the latter part of the night, or the early part of the day. In the unbiassed or natural order of things, this form of fever usually runs its course in ten or fifteen days; but as we have before said, we never yet have been able to satisfy ourselves of the existence of critical days in fever proper—and are forced to believe that this prejudice has arisen from the observance of such a law in the exanthemata, or eruptive fevers, such as measles, small-pox, and the like.

Since this form of fever is the most common, and from the extended theatre of its action interesting a larger portion of our population than the other forms—being common not only to country situations in all climes, but also to cities, and to towns—assailing all ages and all sexes— we have thought proper for these reasons to dwell more upon this than any other link in the chain. Causes: It is partly produced from marsh exhalations, or from breathing an atmosphere impregnated with the exhalations arising from the decaying remains of vegetable and animal substances, and partly from the debilitating influences of excessive fatigue of any kind, the relaxing and debilitating effects of a meagre or unwholesome diet, and partly from the relaxing influence of continued heat on our systems, and partly also from the sudden transitions of temperature. Hence it is that this fever is more common and more fatal as we approach hot climates and low situations, and most prevalent in the hottest seasons of all climates.

This remitting, or continued form of fever, as you may please to call it, though the most common, is the least dangerous—or, in other words, the most manageable form of all the fevers, except that of ague and fever. There are occasional cases, and even occasional seasons, in which it assumes a violent or malignant character from the commencement, or cases and seasons in which, under our best efforts, the disease is apt to run into a low and dangerous grade.

But the causes of these things being for the most part comprehended, and more or less under our own control, might be obviated in due time to save the lives of the sufferers. To explain: the fatal tendencies in most cases arising from mal-practices, such as mal-application of remedial agents, neglect or error in diet, crowding the sick too much together, or the sick and well together, neglect of proper cleanliness, and the want of a free circulation of wholesome air, and a proper attention to the repose of the patient—sleep being as necessary for the well being of the sick as is his food or his physic.

Since fevers, of all kinds and grades, have been known to take life, and are always attended with more or less danger, they should ever be promptly attended to, and, if possible, skilfully managed; for many cases that would yield, under two or three days' judicious management, in the onset of disease, sometimes becomes unmanageable after the lapse of that time.

TREATMENT.

We are well aware of the fact, that the fevers of different seasons, from the peculiar modifying influences of the producing causes, assume different types and different tendencies; that is, that, in some seasons, the congestions or engorgements of the varied organs, necessarily the offspring of the febrile action, are more apt to result in local congestions, while in other seasons they are more prone to degenerate into vitiations, putrescences in the secretions, and, ultimately, to wind up in gangrene or mortifications; such as we witness in some fatal cases of typhoid fevers.

BLOOD-LETTING.

The propriety of abstracting blood will be judged of from the type of the fever, the age and constitution of the patient, and the symptoms present. For example: when cases occur in young and plethoric subjects, and the symptoms indicate much local distress, with a full, free, and active circulation, [of the blood,] then we might expect to practise one or two moderate bleedings to advantage; say, take just blood enough to take off the excess of tension from the pulse. This, we have found, can be achieved by the loss of about three gills, or more, of blood at a bleeding, and should be put in practice in the course of the first two or three days from the attack. The use of this remedy we have confined to particular types, and particular descriptions of cases. If the general bleedings have been neglected at their proper time, or if, after having been duly put in practice, some local pain continues still to distress the patient, we should then seek further relief by the use of cups or blisters applied to the parts most affected; as the judgment of the operator or practitioner may direct.

EMETICS.

In the early stages, and more especially in the onset, or forming stage, of the fever, have we occasionally succeeded in cutting short the disease, by the use of a simple emetic of ipecacuanha, or tartar emetic, (antimonial wine,) giving a preference to the former; followed by the prompt and free use of suitable diluent and diaphoretic drinks, such as flax-seed, sage, chamomile, or black snake-root tea. We ascribe the efficacy of emetics, in such cases, more to the concussion, or revolutionizing effects on the system, whereby the circulation of the blood, and consequent equilibrium of animal heat, and restorative of the secretion of the skin, and other emunctories is effected, than to the mere evacuation of any matter that may take place from the stomach.

In most cases, it is best to pass off the action of the

emetic by such auxiliaries as will unlock the pores of the skin, and thereby mitigate the violence of the fever, such as just above cited; but in those cases where we learn that the patient is in a state of greater or less constipation of the bowels, then we should endeavor to make a gentle impression on the bowels, by the use of a little Epsom salts and gruel, or the senna tea: taking care, at all times, to guard against so great or so hurried an action of these organs as to produce much sensible debility in the patient.

In the use of emetics, as in every other step in the treatment, we should always look well to all the circumstances of the case; not use them where peculiarity or idiosyncracy would forbid, or when the delicacy of the constitution or the already irritated condition of the stomach would oppose it.

CATHARTICS.

While we stand opposed to the practice of attempting the cure of bilious fevers by the exclusive use of cathartics, we are still willing to admit the fact, that such things have been repeatedly done. But we do contend for the practicability of accomplishing the same thing, by a less distressing, less debilitating, and a more than equally safe and short route.

In the early stages of the disease, we approve the use of one or two mercurial cathartics; especially if the stomach be too irritable to bear the administration of the more bulky cathartic drugs. In those cases, we recommend eight or ten grains of calomel, with a half grain of opium, or its equivalent in laudanum or paregoric; or an equivalent of blue mass, in lieu of the calomel, should the patient prefer it. Such doses should or should not be repeated, according to the exigencies of the case. If such dose or doses should fail to operate in due time, then follow it up with a dose of some more common and gentle purgative; such as Epsom salts, castor oil, senna, rhubarb, or such like. So soon as we shall have succeeded in evacuating the stomach and bowels, we consider the patient in a situation to be placed on the use of another class of remedies, viz: the use of tonics and sudorifics. In fact, the author —who has had much experience in the treatment of this form of fever—does not hesitate to commence the treatment by the immediate use of quinine, aided by suitable diaphoretics, at any stage, and without any preparatory depletion.

The extended sales, and the salutary reports from those who have used the author's anti-fever pills, throughout the southern and western States of this Union, in all fevers, and in all stages, go to confirm the facts reported from his own personal experience.

TONICS AND DIAPHORETICS.

Our objections to depending on the depletive practice for the cure of bilious fevers, by repeated pukings or purgings, are, first, because we consider such practices contrary to, or inverting the order of nature; secondly, if experience has taught us that pukes and purges, when used in health, debilitate the individual, and bring on, necessarily, unnatural and almost ungovernable desire for food and for drinks, should it, then, be a matter of surprise that these effects, to a distressing degree, should ensue on the use of such measures in a diseased condition?

We conceive the thirst, now already great from the diseased condition, to be still increased by the increased irritation of the mucous membrane of the stomach and bowels, and as a consequence of the untimely and wanton waste of the fluid elements of the blood.

With this view of the subject, the indications of cure would seem to us to be, to restore the lost balance to the circulation, reinstate the secretions, support the enfeebled system, and allay its morbid irritations.

For the accomplishment of these desirable ends, we have found the judicious and united use of tonic and diaphoretic remedies, aided by well-timed and properly combined opiates, surpassing in efficacy all other means.

Having already stated the time, manner, and circumstances, under which we conceive bleeding, puking or purging, or any one or more of these remedies, necessary at the discretion of the practitioner or attendant, we will now proceed to lay before the reader, in as plain and simple terms as possible, our especial plan of treatment.

We proceed, at once, with the administration of one grain of quinine every two hours, (regardless of fever,) regularly by day and by night, alternating, however, the doses with some suitable diaphoretic, such as the vegetable sweating teas, the Virginia snake root, balm, sage, or the like, the sweet spirit of nitre, the super-carbonates of potash or soda, or a union of the alkalies with some one of the vegetable teas. These drinks may be used either warm or cold, as the patient's appetite may prefer; watching the effects of the diaphoretics, and so regulating the doses or their repetitions, as to procure a slight but general action on the skin, and aiming to maintain such action, without running to any excess. Hence we should suspend the use of the sudorifics whenever there was any danger of excessive perspiration, while we continued that of the tonics. This course of treatment should be continued until a complete crisis, or a marked amelioration is produced. But it not unfrequently happens, that some unpleasant symptom, in connexion with the state of the stomach and bowels, occurs to interrupt the progress of our desired or intended course of treatment, such as a continuance of or a return of sick stomach and vomiting—symptoms constituting what the learned writers have been pleased to call a gastric fever. In such cases we must endeavor, in the first place, to correct or allay such morbid irritation, before we can expect to obtain the benefits of the strictly febrifuge remedies; continuing, however, the use of the quinine, whenever the stomach will retain it.

This will be most effectually done by one or other of the following steps.—Should the patient be troubled with much sense of heat in the stomach, with a casting off of bilious or acid matter, then administer what is called a saline mixture or effervescing draught, as follows: Take of saleratus, bicarbonate of potash, or common salt of tartar, half an ordinary tea-spoon full, fresh lemon juice or vinegar a moderate size table-spoon full. Put the lemon juice or vinegar into a wine-glass, and fill it with water; then add the saleratus, or bicarbonate of potash, made fine: to be immediately taken when added, or drunk in the state of effervescence (or foaming). This dose may be repeated as often as necessary to compose the stomach. Should we fail by this course to obtain the desired relief, then we might make use of any one or more of the following remedies—such as essence of peppermint, the aromatic spirit of hartshorn, the compound spirit of lavender, a few drops of the spirit of turpentine taken in a little cold water or on a lump of sugar, or the use of an opiate portion of morphine, opium, laudanum or paregoric. Of these remedies we have found the opiates the most uniformly successful.

In all cases of irritation of the stomach, more or less benefit may be expected from external applications, such as warm applications, either wet or dry, mustard plasters, blisters, cupping or leeching.

In some instances the irritation of the stomach is kept up or rendered more obstinate from a torpid or inactive state of the bowels; in such cases we should not fail to make some impression on the bowels, either by the use of suitable aperients, or by repeated use of injections.

If, on the other hand, we should have to contend with a wasting from or excessive looseness of the bowels, then we restrain such evacuations by the use of small doses of Dover's powders, paregoric, compound spirit of lavender, tincture of kino, an infusion of the root of the dew-berry or of the common black-berry, or some other suitable astringent, combined or not with a few drops of laudanum, as the presence or absence of pain might indicate.

In all stages of disease and under all circumstances of cases the practitioner should never lose sight of the utility and even importance of any minor considerations of comfort, or of ease, to the patient, such as occasionally bathing the feet, especially at night, in warm water, the application of cold cloths, or cloths saturated with cold water and vinegar, to the head, while there is much excess of heat and pain; or occasionally spunging for the same purpose. But this mode of palliating distress should be practised with caution and with judgment; for if cold applications are made to any part of the body, at or about the period of the decline of fever, or when the patient is too feeble, then unpleasant weakness, restless and sometimes chilly sensations, are the immediate consequence.

We should at all times allow a reasonable indulgence in light and easily digested food, when called for by the natural sensations of the stomach.

Never officiously press upon the patient that which he does not desire, or more or even quite as much as he may desire; we should also pay some regard to the accustomed habits of individuals about taking nourishment, as to point of time—administering our medicines so as to interfere as little as possible with their accustomed periods of eating and sleeping.

In this the reader will not fail to observe an important advantage of our practice over that of the irritating mode of using emetics and cathartics, which are not only irritating to the digestive organs, exhausting to the patient, but at the same time cutting off the regular supply of the continually required new elements of life.

Another very important requisite to the sick is, that they be not molested by unnecessary conversation, or even the presence of unnecessary company. Carefully remove all annoyances of either sight or sound. Give to them all proper opportunities of receiving the refreshing benefits of sleep, and in case of a loss of sleep from diseased or morbid vigilance, or the annoyance of pain, do not hesitate to procure natural rest by the use of a few drops of laudanum, particularly at night, (say twenty or twenty-five drops.)

The strength of the patient, the condition of the tongue, skin and of the pulse, will ever be our surest and best guides as to the indications in the administration of remedies.

The tongue usually covered with a white coat in the commencement of fever, with the progress of symptoms becomes yellow, then brown, and sometimes dark brown, and dry; it sometimes sheds a first coat, and then becomes red, sleek, and glossy, and in extreme cases becomes dry and cracks from a deficiency of its natural secretions.

While these unfavorable symptoms continue to manifest themselves on the tongue, a corresponding want of healthy action exists on the surface of the whole body; the skin continuing for the most part hot and dry, or in a later or lower stage becoming covered with a more or less profuse, sticky, and clammy perspirable matter, with extremities frequently too cool; the pulse during this time becoming weaker with the decline of strength, while its frequency is apt to be increased.

Whenever in the progressive course of a fever the attendant observes that the patient is declining, that is, that he is sinking to a still lower grade, in spite of the use of quinine and the ordinary diaphoretics, whether delirium exists or not, the author has found great benefit result from the use of from three to five grains of camphor, in union with a quarter of a grain of opium, or six or eight drops of laudanum, to be taken once in every six or eight hours, in lieu of the other diaphoretic remedies already recommended; adhering, however, still to the regular use of the quinine, and giving a moderate portion of toddy, milk toddy, or wine and water every two or three hours.

DELIRIUM.—Under our general view of fever we have already given some account of this symptom, as an occasional attendant on fevers. It now becomes necessary to speak of it in this particular form of fever, with a view to the most appropriate mode of combating it. We have already conveyed the idea that that which arrests the fever, arrests its individual manifestations or symptoms. But this symptom has been shown to be partly the effect of the fever proper, and partly the result of a particular organization, or particular temperament. When it occurs in the first stages, it is to be relieved as already directed in the treatment of the first stages of fever, and on the same general principles.

When this symptom occurs in the latter stages of the

fever, then we have found relief from the use of blisters to the back of the neck, and the use of opiates, while in all other respects we continue to treat the case as though no such symptom had occurred.

But a delirium varied and aggravated in its manifestations, and one in which little or no consciousness exists, not unfrequently occurs at a later or in the last stages of the fever. Here it is the result of prostration and irritation; then the indications will be to sustain the vital energies, and to calm its irritations: these indications can be best fulfilled by the use of suitable nourishment, tonics, opiates, blisters, and lastly stimulants, or nourishment, in the form of stimulating drinks, such as wine-whey, milk-toddy, panada, malt liquors, and the like.

There is still another symptom which not unfrequently attends this form of fever, that is, internal irritation, with or without more or less of wasting discharges from the bowels. When such irritation exists without evacuation, that is, when the natural evacuations are retained, then we should procure the necessary and healthy evacuations by the use of laxatives, or in case of much weakness, by injections alone. But if, on the other hand, the patient is wasting from too frequent or too plentiful discharges, then we should endeavor to correct such a state of things by the use of small and repeated doses of opiates and astringents, such as small doses of laudanum, paregoric, tinct. of kino, or any of the vegetable astringent teas. In all those cases of local distress in the bowels, we find warm applications, or applications of mustard, so used as to stimulate without blistering, valuable agents. In proportion to the exhaustion or depression of the patient, is the liability to twitchings of the muscles, a kind of feeble spasmodic action, what the medical writers have called sub sultus tendinum. This symptom is the mere consequence of extreme weakness, and we here draw the attention of the reader to the fact, that he may the more fully see the importance of sustaining his patient in this situation, by all of the means in his power. While we steadily aim to sustain, we should be careful not to overact. This, although a very dangerous symptom, is not necessarily a fatal one.

We have occasionally witnessed cases in which the patient passed no urine for eight or ten days, and still suffered no pain or inconvenience from it; in such cases the secretions are suspended, or the absorbents and exhalants take on an unusual and increased action.

Involuntary discharges by stool or urine occasionally occur in low and protracted cases of fever, and although it is a dangerous symptom or circumstance, it does not necessarily follow that the case must prove fatal.

Let your patients have just so much of the varied stimuli that sustain life, as in the judgment of the practitioner or attendant the organization in its present state can manage, or requires, and no more; and be careful so to time the repetition of your doses as to meet the continually renewed wants of the system.

In case of coldness of the extremities, we should maintain the natural heat by warm applications, or the stimulus of mustard so used as to heat without blistering.

These remarks, applicable to the last stages of disease, will be found equally applicable to all stages.

Before closing the present chapter, we deem it proper to make some general remarks, as an additional guide to whoever may attempt to put in execution our views, viz.: they should ever bear in mind the healthy condition and the healthy needs of the system, and let the object of every step, the use of every agent, be to assist, either directly or indirectly, in bringing back each and every organ of life to the discharge of its healthy function. In all cases, while the sick are able and competent to give us clear and satisfactory responses as to their wants, desires, and sensations; we should never fail patiently to collect such information, and apply it to the benefit of the patient; and in cases of mental alienation, or such torpor of mind as cuts off the aid of the sufferer in explaining himself, then exercise your own judgment on all such other lights as may be brought before you.

As we have been more full and explicit in the detail of remedies, and their application to particular symptoms, in this than in other chapters, for reasons already stated, we have thought proper, here, to remark, that any specifications in the application of remedies to particular symptoms contained in this chapter, that are omitted in other chapters, may, with propriety, be applied to the treatment of like conditions of system occurring in other fevers.

For the doses and modes of administering all the remedies recommended in this chapter, the reader will see chapter XVI.

CHAPTER VIII.

OF CHOLERA INFANTUM, OR, THE PUKING AND PURGING OF CHILDREN; WITH SOME OTHER CONDITIONS OF THE SYSTEM, PECULIAR TO CHILDREN, ATTRIBUTED TO TEETHING AND WORMS.

The author considers cholera infantum as a species of bilious fever, peculiar to children of from six months to two years old. This he infers from the fact, that children of this age are rarely the subjects of either bilious or typhus fevers, but are subject to ague and fever; and from the additional fact, that cholera infantum is much more common in the summer and fall months, and in sickly seasons, when grown persons suffer most from bilious affections.

The reasons for the occurrence of cholera infantum in lieu of bilious fever, would seem to be the peculiar irritability of the stomach and bowels of children at this period of life; being, at this age, more liable to take on unhealthy action, under any circumstances, than at any other period of life. The affections of stomach and bowels which take place in the winter months, being usually slight, and of short duration, while those of the hot seasons are more protracted and more serious in their nature; proving sometimes fatal in a short period, while in other cases they are protracted to many weeks, and even months, until the little sufferers are reduced to mere living skeletons.

The puking and purging in cholera infantum, bears some analogy to the cholera morbus of adults; but is not often so violent, so rapid in its progress, or so fatal in its tendencies—although both diseases may originate from the same, or similar causes.

In cholera infantum, sometimes the vomiting continues without purging, but most generally the purging continues without puking; and it is not uncommon for both symptoms to subside, for six, eight, or ten days, with every appearance of a speedy recovery, and then return or relapse again, after the manner of an intermittent fever. As in other fevers, the violence and the danger of the attack is proportioned to the circumstances of causation and the constitutions of the subjects; hence its greater prevalence and greater fatality in cities, and in warm climates, than in country situations, and in more salubrious climes.

In cholera infantum, as in other fevers, and as in other cases of irritation of the stomach and bowels, the sense of thirst is distressingly great; the patient always desiring more drink than the stomach can digest. In the early part of the disease, the fever is sometimes considerable: the skin is not uniformly hot and dry, as in other fevers; the continued watery wastings from the bowels seem to suppress the natural softness and moisture of the skin.

Towards the close of the disease, and when the patient is much reduced, the hands and feet are apt to be cold; the tongue is apt to be covered with a white fur, and it rarely turns of a dark color. It sometimes becomes sleek and glossy; but when it assumes a dark, or a dark brown aspect, the case is more apt to prove fatal.

TREATMENT.

In the commencement of an attack, we deem it most prudent to suffer the spontaneous evacuations to proceed unmolested, until the stomach and bowels have emptied themselves of their common contents; which is generally accomplished in from six to twelve hours—sometimes in a shorter period. Then we should proceed to allay the irritation of the stomach and bowels, by means of mustard plasters applied over the stomach, so as to stimulate without blistering, and the internal administration of small doses of paregoric, laudanum, essence of peppermint, or some grateful cordial of any kind. Should either the puking or purging run on to excess, then check such discharges—as before directed—by the addition of some astringent, should an unnatural looseness of the bowels require it. We not unfrequently find thin, pale and watery discharges a very obstinate symptom. In such cases, in addition to translating the irritation to the surface of the body, by mustard plasters, we have found it necessary to use repeated doses of some vegetable, astringent drink; and for this purpose we have found no article better than the cold infusion of the root of the common black-berry, or dew-berry. This may be used alone, as a diet-drink, or may be taken in the form of toddy, (with any spirit;) to which might be added an opiate, if the existence of pain required it. Whenever the stomach rejects any of these remedies, the manner of administering should be varied, or, after waiting a reasonable time, the dose again repeated.

In some instances, again, the delicacy of the stomach prohibits the administration of any article. In such cases we should depend on the use of mustard to the stomach and bowels, and the use of anodyne injections; such as a little starch and laudanum, or milk and laudanum.

The teething process being now in progress, no doubt adds much to the increased sensibility and irritability of the child; and whenever any tooth or teeth are coming forward, so as to be marked sources of irritation, then the point of a pen-knife should be passed through the gum, so as to divide the natural envelope of the new tooth.

The coldness of the extremities (so common an attendant) should be obviated by suitable covering, or occasional friction of flour of mustard on the skin.

If the patient does not begin to recover, after using the fore-mentioned remedies for a few days, but continues to be out of tone, or suffering from a feverish state, or seems weak and exhausted, then commence with suitable doses of quinine; and repeat every two or three hours, until there is a solution of diseased action—a complete crisis. Then lengthen the interval between doses to two or three doses a day, and continue its use in this way until the little patient is reinstated in health and strength. [For medicine and doses see chapter XVI.]

During the continuance of the warmer season, children are very liable to relapses. This can most effectually be guarded against by seeking a purer atmosphere; attention to cleanliness, diet, and exercise.

OF TEETHING AND OF WORMS.

It is a popular doctrine with the profession, and consequently with the community at large, the latter never having taken on themselves the trouble to think about medicine or diseases, excepting through the medium of their family doctors, (who are not always sages,) that teething, or worms, or both, are causes of cholera infantum. Now while we oppose this idea, we are willing to see in them sources of irritation worthy to be noticed and attended to.

The growth of teeth is as natural and as necessary as the growth of bones, muscles, or nerves, and we presume are produced by the same or similar processes; if so, why not contend that these things are sources of disease? The only appreciable difference would seem to us to be, that the one has a marked crisis, the other not; that is, the period at which the tooth makes its exit from the gum. Now this lasts but a few days, while the cholera infantum is liable to continue during the whole warm season. But the opposition will say that the teething still continues too. To this we reply, that the cholera infantum does not commence in the winter season, or even run into the winter months, although the teething process is still going on, regardless of the changes of the seasons: moreover, there are very many children who get their teeth without the slightest complaint or indisposition of any kind; particularly those who pass through the teething process while very young.

Again, we hear no complaint about the stomach and bowels attendant on the shedding of teeth, when there is not only a new growth in progress, but the additional irritation of casting off the old ones.

We readily admit the greater liability of children to disease, and to death, during the first two years of existence, than at any other equivalent of time; for the existence of this truth, many other reasons might be added to that of teething and worms, such as nursing, diet, atmospheric circumstances, and the like.

WORMS.

As to the presence of worms, we know them frequently to exist, and sometimes in considerable numbers, in children apparently in sound and vigorous health. As to the prime origin or mode of propagating this family of vermin, it is a matter still in obscurity. The weight of testimony on this subject is in favor of the idea of a spontaneous generation in the human intestines; and the circumstances of life most favorable to such generations would seem to be youth, excessive feeding, and more especially the use of unwholesome and indigestible food, or whatever other causes that may tend to derange the functions of digestion or of assimilation.

With this view of the subject we are led to the belief that the existence of worms is more frequently a result than a cause of disease. But that when they have been generated, and more especially when they exist in great numbers, that they then become an additional cause of irritation, emaciation, and of febrile disease, and should not only be promptly expelled by the use of suitable vermifuges, but that the patient should afterwards be placed on the use of such remedies as would most effectually prevent their return or regeneration.

The symptoms ascribed to, and that possibly may be attendant on worms in children, are almost as numerous, and very much resembling the symptoms of many other diseases to which they are subject. Therefore it is impossible to discriminate them, with absolute certainty, from the symptoms of many other indispositions. This must be left to the discretion of the practitioner or attendant·

and these facts afford us an additional proof of the unity of disease.

SYMPTOMS.

The presence of worms is generally indicated by variableness of appetite, fœtor of the breath, restlessness and grinding of the teeth in the sleep, picking of the nose, or swelling of the upper lip, more or less of tumefaction of the belly, disturbance of the bowels, pain or uneasy sensations about the navel, febrile distress, and lastly, the passing of worms. When any or all of these signs point to the presence of worms, we should administer vermifuges, such as a tea of the root of the Spigelia or Carolina pink-root; one, two, or more grains of calomel, according to the age of the patient, should be administered every second morning for two doses; or the oil of wormseed two or three times per day for some days in succession; or a few drops of the spirit of turpentine with a little sugar and water two or three times per day. Should there exist a costive state of the bowels while using the worm medicines, then you should purge gently with a little senna tea, castor oil, or a dose of calomel; provided that article has not yet been used.

In every case of worms, after having succeeded in expelling them, the patient should be placed on the use of some bitter tonic, until restored to good health and to good digestion. For this purpose we know of nothing preferable to the use of suitable doses of quinine. In truth, we have reason to believe that it is itself a good vermifuge, either from its bitter principle or its tonic effects on the system. The tonic preparations of iron are also well suited to such cases. For particulars as to remedies and their doses, the reader will see chap. 16.

CHAPTER IX.

YELLOW FEVER.

"Nous perdrions une grande partie le notre savoir, si nous pouvions 'etre delivrie tout a coup de tous nos erreurs."—PIBRAC.

The increase of knowledge is not like that of other things; being often accompanied by a considerable diminution in bulk.

DESCRIPTION.—According to our classification of fevers this is the lowest grade and most malignant type of bilious diseases. It is to common bilious fever what cold plague or spotted fever is to typhus or nervous fever, and might with propriety be called the typhoid bilious fever of cities and of southern climes, since it never appears in high latitudes, except in hot seasons and in crowded, illy ventilated and filthy places; and even in southern and tropical regions its ravages are checked by the coming on of the colder seasons of the year. It is more violent in its attacks, more rapid in its progress, and more putrescent and fatal in its tendency, than any other form of bilious fever.

CAUSES.

The concentrated virus of marsh exhalations, combined with the exhalations from human exuviæ, brought into action upon systems enfeebled by any or all of the vices of civic life; that is to say, the debilitating and deranging effects resulting from a violation of organic laws, aided by the continued and relaxing influences of heat; or, in other words, the external causes are, the combined influence of heat with a peculiar vitiation of atmosphere—while the internal causes are violations of organic laws.

The united effects of these two classes of modifying causes are to debilitate, to overcome, to cripple and derange the functional action of the whole man, in brain, nerves, muscles, and all the glandular tissues. Hence we see such rapid tendencies in the secretions to vitiations and putrescencies—while in the solids, particularly in the stomach and bowels, there is a rapid running into gangrene and mortification, as is evinced by the black and putrid matters discharged from them, and the speedy triumphs of death and decomposition that we are occasionally called to witness.

We are aware that a prejudice exists, not only in the minds of the populace but of the profession, yea, even among the anointed of the schools, that all of these symptoms and destructive tendencies are ascribable, either to the quantity or quality of the bile, or both.—(Poor liver, it is really distressing to think of the many false charges brought up against thee.) If the mere abundance or vitiation of the secretions of the liver could work such rapid and fatal changes, how is it that jaundice, (evidently as much a bilious affection as yellow fever,) which is common to all climates and to all seasons, is so seldom fatal? When it occurs in constitutions reasonably good, it rarely produces even fever; although the bile is freely diffused over and through the whole system, the patient in many instances is scarcely conscious of being diseased, except from the color of the skin.

SYMPTOMS.

The attack of yellow fever is, in most particulars, like that of other fevers. It is usually ushered in by sensations of lassitude and weakness, a stiffness or soreness of the muscles, pain of the head, back and limbs, generally accompanied by some degree of chilliness; these precursors are soon succeeded by increased pain of the head and frontal sinuses, giddiness or dizziness, flushings of the face, a sense of fullness in the eye-balls, with an expression of distress in the countenance; the eyes red and suffused with tears, a general sense of debility with thirst, either great restlessness with signs of delirium, or a tendency to lethargy; urine high colored, scanty and turbid; perspiration irregular, interrupted and diminished; pulse irregular, either too hurried or too slow, full, fretful and hobbling, often giving the delusive feeling of increased force, seldom strictly tense; tongue covered with a whitish mucous coat; great irritability of stomach, with nausea and vomiting of bilious matter; bowels usually bound, epigastrium (pit of the stomach) tender on pressure.

In the course of twenty-four or thirty-six hours, or by the close of the first paroxysm, the eyes usually become of a deep yellow, which readily spreads over the face, neck, breast, and finally the whole body. The foregoing symptoms, in a greater or less degree, usually attend on the first stage of the disease, and there is rarely an abatement of symptoms, until the disease has gone through the first stage or first paroxysm, which generally lasts from twenty-four to forty-eight hours, when an evident remission takes place, sometimes with such marked amelioration of symptoms as to induce the patient to think himself almost well or out of danger. But a speedy recurrence of the paroxysm, with an aggravation of symptoms, soon convinces him of his error.

As the disease advances, symptoms more and more indicative of a fatal termination manifest themselves; the patient's strength continues to decline, the skin becomes of a deeper and a darker hue, patches of livid spots begin to be observable on different parts of the body, delirium increases, the secretions begin to show signs of putrescency, the tongue becomes dark and dry, the teeth are encrusted with a dark matter, the breath is fœtid, hickups ensue, hœmorrages are apt to break forth from the mouth, nostrils or elsewhere, dark fœtid and involuntary discharges take place from the bowels, the pulse sinks, and death quickly closes the scene. Such are the ordinary displays in those cases which terminate speedily in death.

In this fever, as in all fevers proper, there are no marked critical days—the duration of disease, whether terminating favorably or otherwise, will be in proportion to the violence of the causes and the constitutions of the subjects of disease. Being a malignant disease, it usually runs its course in from two to five or seven days; recoveries from cases protracted beyond this period are, for the most part, tardy and imperfect, the patients suffering more or less from indigestion, the necessary result of injuries sustained by the stomach during the continuance of the disease.

If the spring of action which has induced us to write these pages had been either pecuniary gain or popular applause, then should we have consulted the public will, the popular prejudice, courted the smiles of those who occupy the high places of human ordination, submitted to the prejudices, opinions and practices, of distinguished cotemporaries, and invoked the spirits of the illustrious dead; but being impelled by an unbiassed love of truth, and an ardor for usefulness, we have been forced to deviate materially from such a course.

Believing, as we do, that truth is the exclusive property of no man, and that the terminus of thought, either in this or in any other department of human research, has not yet been reached, and that, when reached and explained, it will be found to rest on simple, uniform, and eternal laws, we have ventured to raise a voice, if not in opposition, certainly not in accordance with any of our illustrious predecessors. We shall endeavor to offer a more plain and simple view, in the treatment of this disease, than any heretofore presented, and one, too, which we conceive to be more strictly calculated to counteract the virus of the disease; and that, too, in accordance with the natural laws of life.

In consulting the pages of medical history, we find the weight of authority decidedly in favor of the depletive practice; at least, since the days of the immortal Rush. We say immortal, because to him are we indebted, in a great measure, for the demonstration of its domestic origin; to him are we indebted for some of the clearest lights on the subject of contagion; also, for the earliest, the freeest, and the fullest experiments in the depletive practices.

When the yellow fever made its appearance in Philadelphia, in 1793, Dr. Rush seems to have been much at a loss as to what course of treatment he should pursue. In this state of mind, he sought the experience of a Dr. Stevens.—We will give his report, in his own words:

"Perplexed and distressed by my want of success in the

treatment of this fever, I waited upon Dr. Stevens, an eminent and worthy physician from St. Croix, who happened, then, to be in our city, and asked for such advice and information upon the subject of the disease, as his extensive practice in the West Indies would naturally suggest. He politely informed me, that he had long ago laid aside evacuations of all kinds in the yellow fever: that they had been found to be hurtful; and that the disease yielded more readily to bark, wine, and, above all, to the use of the cold bath.

"He advised the bark to be given in large quantities, by way of clyster as well as in the usual way; and he informed me of the manner in which the cold bath should be used, so as to derive the greatest benefit from it. This mode of treating the yellow fever appeared to be reasonable. I had used bark, in the manner he recommended it, in several cases of sporadic yellow fever, with success, in former years. I had, moreover, the authority of several other physicians of reputation in its favor. Dr. Cleghorn tells us, that he sometimes gave the bark when the bowels were full of vicious humors. 'These humors,' he says, 'are produced by the fault of the circulation. The bark, by bracing the solids, enables them to throw off the excrementitious fluids by the proper emunctories.'

"I began the use of Dr. Stevens' remedies the next day after my interview with him, with great confidence of their success. I prescribed bark in large quantities. In one case I ordered it to be injected into the bowels every four hours. I directed buckets full of cold water to be thrown frequently upon my patients. The bark was offensive to the stomach, or rejected by it, in every case in which I prescribed it. The cold bath was grateful, and produced relief in several cases, by inducing a moisture on the skin. For a while, I had hope of benefit to my patients from the use of these remedies; but in a few days I was distressed to find they were not more effectual than those I had previously used. Three out of four of my patients died; to whom the cold bath was administered, in addition to the tonic remedies before mentioned." [R. W. vol. ii., p. 125.]

The doctor, being not pleased with the result of his practice and limited experiments, under the instructions of Dr. Stevens, we find him, in the course of a very few days, running upon the opposite extreme. His mind first settles down on the propriety of free and repeated purgings. His words are:

"One dose was sometimes sufficient to open the bowels, but from two to six were often necessary for that purpose; more especially as part of them were frequently rejected by the stomach. I did not observe any inconvenience from the vomiting which was excited by the jalap. It was always without that straining which was produced by emetics; and it served to discharge bile when it was lodged in the stomach. Nor did I rest the discharge of the contents of the bowels on the issue of one cleansing on the first day. There is, in all bilious fevers, a reproduction of morbid bile as fast as it is discharged: I therefore gave a purge every day, while the fever continued. I used castor-oil, salts, cremor tartar, and rhubarb, (after the mercurial purges had performed their office,) according to the inclination of my patients, in all those cases where the bowels were easily moved; but where this was not the case, I gave a single dose of calomel and jalap every day. Strong as this purge may be supposed to be, it was often ineffectual; more especially after the 20th of September, when the bowels became more obstinately constipated. To supply the place of the jalap, I now added gamboge to the calomel. Two grains and a half of each, made into a pill, were given to an adult every six hours, until they procured four or five stools." [R. W., vol. ii., p. 133.]

The doctor, we have said, on abandoning the tonic plan of treatment, suggested by Dr. Stevens, immediately runs upon the opposite extreme: he now not only practises free and continued purgings, but he has become equally bold in the use of his lancet. The words of the immortal sage are:

"In determining the quantity of blood to be drawn, I was governed by the state of the pulse, and the temperature of the weather. In the beginning of September, I

found one or two moderate bleedings sufficient to subdue the fever; but in proportion as the system rose, by the diminution of the stimulus of heat, and the fever put on more visible signs of inflammatory diathesis, more frequent bleedings became necessary. I bled many patients twice, and a few three times a day. I preferred frequent and small, to large bleedings, in the month of September; but towards the height and close of the epidemic, I saw no inconvenience from the loss of a pint, and even twenty ounces of blood at a time. I drew from many persons seventy and eighty ounces in five days, and from a few a much larger quantity. Mr. Gribble, cedar cooper, in Front street, lost, by ten bleedings, a hundred ounces of blood; Mr. George, a carter, in North street, lost about the same quantity in five bleedings; and Mr. Peter Meerken, one hundred and fourteen ounces in five days. In the last of the above persons, the quantity taken was determined by weight. Mr. Foy, blacksmith, near Dock street, was eight times bled, in the course of seven days. The quantity taken from him was about a hundred ounces. The blood, in all these cases, was dense, and in the last very sizy. They were all attended in the month of October, and chiefly by my pupil, Mr. Fisher: and they were all, years, afterwards, living and healthy instances of the efficacy of copious blood-letting, and of the intrepidity and judgment of this young physician." [See Rush's Works, vol. ii., page 147.]

Now that we have patiently followed the doctor through some of his transitions of opinion, and witnessed the processes by which he has been delivered of his errors, we will next call the attention of the reader to some of the earliest phenomena of Rush and the fever.

In vol. ii., page 42, he says: "On the 19th of this month (meaning August) I was requested to visit the wife of Mr. Peter La Maigre, in Water street between Arch and Race streets, in consultation with Dr. Faulke and Dr. Hodge. I found her in the last stage of a highly bilious fever. She vomited constantly, and complained of great heat and burning in her stomach. The most powerful

cordials and tonics were prescribed, but to no purpose. She died on the evening of the next day. The origin of this fever was discovered to me at the same time, from the account which Dr. Faulke gave me of a quantity of damaged coffee which had been thrown upon Ball's wharf and in the adjoining dock on the 24th of July, nearly in a line with Mr. Le Maigre's house, and which had putrified there, to the great annoyance of the whole neighbourhood. After this consultation I was soon able to trace all of the cases of fever which I have mentioned to this cause."

Again, page 47, he says: "From a conviction that the disease originated in the putrid exhalations from the damaged coffee, I published in the American Daily Advertiser, of August 29th, a short address to the citizens of Philadelphia, with a view of directing public attention to the spot where the coffee lay, and thereby of checking the progress of the fever as far as it was continued by the original cause."

"The seeds of the fever, when received into the body, were generally excited into action in a few days. I met with several cases in which they acted so as to produce a fever on the same day in which they were received into the system, and I heard of two cases in which they excited sickness, fainting, and fever within one hour after the persons were exposed to them. I met with no instance in which there was a longer interval than sixteen days between their being received into the body and the production of the disease.

"This poison acted differently in different constitutions, according to previous habits, to the degrees of predisposing debility, or to the quantity and concentration of the miasmata which had been received into the body."

The doctor further tells us that, in addition to the poisoned state of the atmosphere, the fever was excited by the following causes, acting directly or indirectly upon the system. (See pages 42, 48, 50, and 51, Rush's Works.)

"First. Great labor, or exercise of body or mind, in walking, riding, watching, or the like.

"Second. Heat from every cause, but more especially

the heat of the sun, was a very common exciting cause of the disease.

"Third. Intemperance in eating or drinking.

"Fourth. Fear. In many people the disease was excited by a sudden paroxysm of fear.

"Fifth. Grief; sixth, cold; seventh, sleep; eighth, immoderate evacuations."

Under all these acknowledged predisposing causes to debilitate the body and mind, Dr. Rush bleeds and purges repeatedly and profusely.

If the noxious effluvia (call it by what name you please) emanating from putrifying vegetable and animal matters, such as the damaged coffee thrown upon Ball's wharf in Philadelphia, be the real cause and poison that produces yellow fever, then is it most rational to expect to relieve the persons infected with such poison, by copious and repeated bleedings and purgings, or to hunt a proper antidote to such poison? But the opposition will say that so sudden are the attacks, so rapid the progress of disease towards a fatal issue, that less efficient and more tardy remedies would be of no avail, because individuals become the subjects of disease from one or more days' exposure to the infected atmosphere, or even a few hours, and frequently become its victims in two or three days from the period of the attack.

It has been our fate to witness the effects of poisons (of many kinds and introduced in the many ways) upon the animal economy.

We have seen individuals suddenly thrown into fevers, into vomitings, into cramps, convulsions, syncope or fainting, from breathing for a time mephitic gases of different kinds, such as what the miners and well-diggers call damps or damp airs; we have seen individuals for a time divested of all the ordinary signs of life, yet we have never relied on bleeding and purging for the restoration of such persons. We have been called to witness the effects of animal poisons, such as the bite of spiders and venomous serpents. We have witnessed the rapid tumefaction (the sudden inflammation if you prefer the expression) the spasms, heard the oft repeated cries of pain, observed the tears of woe, yet still we have not relied on bleeding and purging for the relief of such cases; and even when vegetable, animal, or mineral poisons have been just swallowed, we have not relied more on evacuating remedies than the use of such antidotes as are known to neutralize or counteract the deleterious properties of the particular poisons taken. Why then should we place our chief reliance upon these measures in cases of putrid or malignant fevers?

Doctor Rush, in the first cases of the epidemic yellow fever of 1793, treated them with the depletive remedies, viz.: blood-letting and purging with calomel, salts, cream of tartar. See his works, page 41, vol. ii.

Why he abandoned that course he does not say; but we find him shortly afterwards experimenting with ipecacuanha, bark, wine, brandy, aromatics, blisters, finally blankets dipped in warm vinegar and frictions of mercurial ointment on the right side. See his works, vol. ii. p. 125.

Next we find him asking counsel of Dr. Stevens, an eminent physician from St. Croix.

He recommended the free use of bark, wine, and the cold bath. This mode of treating the yellow fever appeared reasonable to the Doctor; he had used bark in the manner recommended in several cases of sporadic yellow fever, with success in former years. In fact, the Doctor was so well pleased with the suggestion of Dr. Stevens, that he proceeded to put his practice in execution the very next day.

Now to you it may seem strange that Rush should so soon change his opinion again, while Dr. Stevens, so far as we know and believe, never did. It may be, that there is as much in the skill and judgment with which scientific labors are executed, as in the powers of intellect in which the truths of science are conceived.

In his first experiments with the tonic and stimulating practice, (see his works, vol. 2, p. 125,) ten out of thirteen patients died. In his second experiments, now aided by the experience of Dr. Stevens of St. Croix, he lost only three out of four—that is a very small fraction less. To us it is not a matter of surprise that he should have failed in both experiments, for the reason, that in every thing that he said, in every thing that he did, he displayed too much of the ultra. In his first experiments he stimulated to excess, he physiced without judgment. From his own words we have the right to infer that he expected to carry his point by storm. In his second experiment, or his effort to execute the counsel of Dr. Stevens, he failed, because he did not in truth, (from the clear inference of his own words,) try the experiment; he paid no attention to the state of his patient's stomach;—see the consequences: " The bark was offensive to the stomach, or rejected by it, in every case in which I prescribed it." We have been taught to believe, that to read and not to understand is not to read at all. The cold bath, a most potent agent either for good or for evil, seems to have been too carelessly directed.

His words are: " I directed buckets of cold water to be thrown frequently on my patients." What good could any one expect from a remedy of doubtful efficacy at most, under such vague instructions?

The Doctor, finding himself " baffled in every attempt to stop the ravages of this fever," again betook himself to intense study. " He ransacked his library, and pored over every book that treated of yellow fever." Finally, he overhauled a manuscript that had been placed in his hands by Dr. Franklin a short time before his death. This paper and the aid of Dr. Mitchell resulted in leading him to return again to the depletive, particularly the purgative practice. Presently we see him enraptured with the virtues of calomel and jalap; doses of ten and ten are now distributed in a wholesale manner throughout the city; indeed, so great is his confidence in the purgative remedies, that he directs his patients to be purged every day while the fever lasted.

His next remedy is the lancet; he bled " many patients twice, and a few three times a day;" he " preferred frequent and small to large bleedings, in the month of September," "but towards the height and close of the epidemic" he "saw no inconvenience from the loss of a pint, and even twenty ounces of blood at a time; he drew from many persons seventy and eighty ounces in five days, and from a few a much larger quantity."

We have thought fit to dwell on this bold feature in Rush's practice, to show that he was in this, as in all other notable thoughts and acts of his life, an ultra.

We have set out with the desire to pursue strictly the philosophic walks; we have condemned all officious intermeddlings, and have taken the position that it is better to do nothing than to do wrong; that the business of the physician is to study nature's laws, and to act conformably thereto; to remove obstacles, and to offer facilities, as the circumstances might indicate; in other words, to observe and to assist nature, when and where we understand the language of her wants; but never to officiously trespass on her reserved and sovereign rights. But the Dr. says that "he took the cure entirely out of nature's hands." Rush's Works, vol. 2, p. 145.

Now, expressions like these to our ears savors too strongly of ultraism, of egotism; such individuals would not scruple to violate a natural law to maintain or establish one of his own ordination.

We have been induced to dwell thus minutely upon the treatment of yellow fever, for the reason that we are well aware, not only of the popular prejudices that have been created, and that still stand opposed to us, but that the names of distinguished living writers, men high in office, individuals whose names have gone abroad and whose words have been received as the oracles of truth, are still actors on the stage of usefulness, the theatre of doctors.

Dr. James Johnson, of London, who, in our humble opinion, is one of the soundest medical philosophers now living, the classical and talented author of "Tropical Climates," "Civic Life," "Change of Air," and some other works of equal celebrity, tells us, (see his "Tropical Climates," vol. 2, p. 338,) under the signature of Archibald

Robertson, Member of the Royal Medical Society of Edinburgh,) as follows:

"Of the general treatment of the epidemic fever I come next to speak. Regarding this disease to be, to all practical intents and purposes, inflammatory, and the affection of the head to be primary and essential, which is evinced by headach, intolerantia lucis, and red eyes, occurring as the earliest symptoms—for the eye is here generally an index of the state of the brain, in the same manner as the tongue is of the state of the stomach—I have never hesitated to push evacuations to the utmost. Bleeding from the arm or frontal branch of the temporal artery was always my first step; and large and repeated blood-lettings during the early stage (the earlier the better) I consider the great palladium of the patient's safety. During the first twelve hours of the disease I have generally drawn from fifty to sixty ounces; but there can be no general rule as to how many ounces should be taken; we ought to bleed to syncope, and bleed repeatedly, in order to break the morbid association of the symptoms, and induce a speedy remission: for I am convinced, that it is not only by its unloading the vessels, but by the shock, (I cannot express it in philosophical language,) which it gives to the whole system, nervous as well as vascular, that blood-letting affords the magical relief I have so often witnessed; it is also chiefly by the inexplicable changes implied in the word shock, that cold effusion operates advantageously; for in tropical climates, where the temperature of sea-water is generally from 80 to 82, its refrigerating power must be much abated.

"The state of the pulse is less to be regarded than the urgency of the other symptoms: the latter often imperiously demand renewed depletion, even when the former is thready, spreading, or undulating; and their demand must be complied with at all hazards. In a disease like this, where the danger is frequently imminent in twelve or fifteen hours, it is often amazing how much its apparent character may be altered by active depletion."

Again, he says:

"It is an Herculean disease, and without that almost omnipotent remedy, the lancet, we might be said to encounter it unarmed; for all other means are but of secondary force."

"It requires all the vigor and activity imaginable, else it will gain ground on us with rapid strides. It is indispensable to bleed, again and again: this is the mainstay—the sheet anchor of hope. Without it, many, very many, must infallibly be lost. Would I could say, that by it all are saved!"

The same writer further remarks—page 341:

"Purging,—free purging,—I have not hitherto mentioned, the necessity being so much a matter of course. A stimulus ought to be kept up constantly on the bowels, if with no other view than to relieve the head."

We have contended that the inflammation of fevers,—the ideal phantom, so much feared and so desperately combated by the blood-letters and the purgers,—whenever and wherever it occurred, was a consequence of the fever, and not its cause; and a consequence too frequently resulting from mal-practices, mal-management, or neglect. But some of our adversaries hold out the idea that it is the cause; others, that it is the direct effect, the direct tendency of the fever to result in inflammation, and thus to produce death. But, unfortunately for such reasoners, we find that such views are but illy sustained, even by their own autopsies, to which they are fond to make appeals.

Let us see what this said Dr. Robertson has to say—p. 335, vol. ii., Johnston's Tropical Climates:

"On examining the stomach," (which he says, elsewhere, is, from the first, highly irritable, and so continues,) "I found the vessels on its inner coat much more conspicuous than natural, and filled with dark, grumous blood; but without any distinct traces of acute inflammation. In the lungs, and other viscera of the thorax and abdomen, there were no appearance of inflammation whatever, and none of congestion, save such as might readily be accounted for by venous gravitation.

"In the brain or its membranes I found few traces of

found one or two moderate bleedings sufficient to subdue the fever; but in proportion as the system rose, by the diminution of the stimulus of heat, and the fever put on more visible signs of inflammatory diathesis, more frequent bleedings became necessary. I bled many patients twice, and a few three times a day. I preferred frequent and small, to large bleedings, in the month of September; but towards the height and close of the epidemic, I saw no inconvenience from the loss of a pint, and even twenty ounces of blood at a time. I drew from many persons seventy and eighty ounces in five days, and from a few a much larger quantity. Mr. Gribble, cedar cooper, in Front street, lost, by ten bleedings, a hundred ounces of blood; Mr. George, a carter, in North street, lost about the same quantity in five bleedings; and Mr. Peter Meerken, one hundred and fourteen ounces in five days. In the last of the above persons, the quantity taken was determined by weight. Mr. Foy, blacksmith, near Dock street, was eight times bled, in the course of seven days. The quantity taken from him was about a hundred ounces. The blood, in all these cases, was dense, and in the last very sizy. They were all attended in the month of October, and chiefly by my pupil, Mr. Fisher: and they were all, years, afterwards, living and healthy instances of the efficacy of copious blood-letting, and of the intrepidity and judgment of this young physician." [See Rush's Works, vol. ii., page 147.]

Now that we have patiently followed the doctor through some of his transitions of opinion, and witnessed the processes by which he has been delivered of his errors, we will next call the attention of the reader to some of the earliest phenomena of Rush and the fever.

In vol. ii., page 42, he says: "On the 19th of this month (meaning August) I was requested to visit the wife of Mr. Peter La Maigre, in Water street between Arch and Race streets, in consultation with Dr. Faulke and Dr. Hodge. I found her in the last stage of a highly bilious fever. She vomited constantly, and complained of great heat and burning in her stomach. The most powerful

cordials and tonics were prescribed, but to no purpose. She died on the evening of the next day. The origin of this fever was discovered to me at the same time, from the account which Dr. Faulke gave me of a quantity of damaged coffee which had been thrown upon Ball's wharf and in the adjoining dock on the 24th of July, nearly in a line with Mr. Le Maigre's house, and which had putrified there, to the great annoyance of the whole neighbourhood. After this consultation I was soon able to trace all of the cases of fever which I have mentioned to this cause."

Again, page 47, he says: "From a conviction that the disease originated in the putrid exhalations from the damaged coffee, I published in the American Daily Advertiser, of August 29th, a short address to the citizens of Philadelphia, with a view of directing public attention to the spot where the coffee lay, and thereby of checking the progress of the fever as far as it was continued by the original cause."

"The seeds of the fever, when received into the body, were generally excited into action in a few days. I met with several cases in which they acted so as to produce a fever on the same day in which they were received into the system, and I heard of two cases in which they excited sickness, fainting, and fever within one hour after the persons were exposed to them. I met with no instance in which there was a longer interval than sixteen days between their being received into the body and the production of the disease.

"This poison acted differently in different constitutions, according to previous habits, to the degrees of predisposing debility, or to the quantity and concentration of the miasmata which had been received into the body."

The doctor further tells us that, in addition to the poisoned state of the atmosphere, the fever was excited by the following causes, acting directly or indirectly upon the system. (See pages 42, 48, 50, and 51, Rush's Works.)

"First. Great labor, or exercise of body or mind, in walking, riding, watching, or the like.

"Second. Heat from every cause, but more especially

found one or two moderate bleedings sufficient to subdue the fever; but in proportion as the system rose, by the diminution of the stimulus of heat, and the fever put on more visible signs of inflammatory diathesis, more frequent bleedings became necessary. I bled many patients twice, and a few three times a day. I preferred frequent and small, to large bleedings, in the month of September; but towards the height and close of the epidemic, I saw no inconvenience from the loss of a pint, and even twenty ounces of blood at a time. I drew from many persons seventy and eighty ounces in five days, and from a few a much larger quantity. Mr. Gribble, cedar cooper, in Front street, lost, by ten bleedings, a hundred ounces of blood; Mr. George, a carter, in North street, lost about the same quantity in five bleedings; and Mr. Peter Meerken, one hundred and fourteen ounces in five days. In the last of the above persons, the quantity taken was determined by weight. Mr. Foy, blacksmith, near Dock street, was eight times bled, in the course of seven days. The quantity taken from him was about a hundred ounces. The blood, in all these cases, was dense, and in the last very sizy. They were all attended in the month of October, and chiefly by my pupil, Mr. Fisher: and they were all, years, afterwards, living and healthy instances of the efficacy of copious blood-letting, and of the intrepidity and judgment of this young physician." [See Rush's Works, vol. ii., page 147.]

Now that we have patiently followed the doctor through some of his transitions of opinion, and witnessed the processes by which he has been delivered of his errors, we will next call the attention of the reader to some of the earliest phenomena of Rush and the fever.

In vol. ii., page 42, he says: "On the 19th of this month (meaning August) I was requested to visit the wife of Mr. Peter La Maigre, in Water street between Arch and Race streets, in consultation with Dr. Faulke and Dr. Hodge. I found her in the last stage of a highly bilious fever. She vomited constantly, and complained of great heat and burning in her stomach. The most powerful

cordials and tonics were prescribed, but to no purpose. She died on the evening of the next day. The origin of this fever was discovered to me at the same time, from the account which Dr. Faulke gave me of a quantity of damaged coffee which had been thrown upon Ball's wharf and in the adjoining dock on the 24th of July, nearly in a line with Mr. Le Maigre's house, and which had putrified there, to the great annoyance of the whole neighbourhood. After this consultation I was soon able to trace all of the cases of fever which I have mentioned to this cause."

Again, page 47, he says: " From a conviction that the disease originated in the putrid exhalations from the damaged coffee, I published in the American Daily Advertiser, of August 29th, a short address to the citizens of Philadelphia, with a view of directing public attention to the spot where the coffee lay, and thereby of checking the progress of the fever as far as it was continued by the original cause."

" The seeds of the fever, when received into the body, were generally excited into action in a few days. I met with several cases in which they acted so as to produce a fever on the same day in which they were received into the system, and I heard of two cases in which they excited sickness, fainting, and fever within one hour after the persons were exposed to them. I met with no instance in which there was a longer interval than sixteen days between their being received into the body and the production of the disease.

" This poison acted differently in different constitutions, according to previous habits, to the degrees of predisposing debility, or to the quantity and concentration of the miasmata which had been received into the body."

The doctor further tells us that, in addition to the poisoned state of the atmosphere, the fever was excited by the following causes, acting directly or indirectly upon the system. (See pages 42, 48, 50, and 51, Rush's Works.)

" First. Great labor, or exercise of body or mind, in walking, riding, watching, or the like.

" Second. Heat from every cause, but more especially

the cathartics, however, fail to perform their office well on the first two days, the disease advances steadily, threatening at every step to some vital organ. Under these circumstances we must resort to bleeding again and again, and redouble our efforts to excite the peristaltic action of the bowels. After the second day, blisters may be employed with great advantage to arrest vomiting (which is frequently, though not universally, a distressing symptom,) to releive gastric pain, or to act as a revulsion of cerebral excitement. The therapeutic means detailed, in connexion with diluents and cold ablutions, constitute the main and perhaps the only remedies required in this fever.

"Tonics, in most cases, are not necessary; none but the mildest, such as camomile infusion, can be administered with advantage; the more powerful, such as sulphate of quinine, are absolutely inadmissible.* This disease runs its course in a short time, either proving fatal in a few days by a concentration of its forces on some organ, or

---

* The reasons why the virtues and the proper uses of quinine have been so tardy in arriving at a full and complete development, we conceive to be the following, viz: In the first place, in the ealier periods of its introduction into practice, physicians could not well have attained to a knowledge of its full virtues, by reason of the bulk of the inert cortical mass with which it was encumbered, causing it to disagree with the stomach, they not having learned to extract its salts, the quinine in which its virtues are concentrated. Secondly, because few, very few, even in our own time, seem to have clear ideas of the properties of, or the modus operandi of strictly tonic remedies. They are for the most part disposed to associate ideas of a stimulating or inflaming nature with all the tonic remedies, and especially that of quinine.

Thirdly, their applications of it to practice under such prejudices have restricted its use exclusively to the periods of remission and of intermission.

Some have erred in using doses too small or at intervals too long, while others again have run into the opposite extreme. Some again may have been disappointed, from the unfavorable condition of the patients on whom their experiments were made. One thing certainly is passingly strange; that is, that, while all agree in ascribing to the drug febrifuge properties, scarcely any are willing to administer it while there is the slightest fever.

being itself vanquished on the fifth or seventh day. Having once yielded, the disease seldom renews the conflict."

The surgeon's opinions and practices in the use of quinine, stand in direct opposition to our own. He even thinks quinine inadmissible in the convalescence from the fever, while we use it in every stage. He must think that it favors inflammation or aggravates fever, while our experience gives to it opposite effects. We ascribe to it febrifuge, antiseptic, and tonic virtues: he places great reliance upon the supervention of ptyalism, (salivation,) which we never desire to witness.

Before we venture to give our personal views upon this intricate and unsettled subject, we have thought fit, first, to introduce some of the adverse opinions that have already found their way to the public eye. In Boisseau's admirable treatise on fevers, we have found the following quotation from the experience of M. Bally:

"The same author declares, that emetics have seldom succeeded in America. An unhappy experience in a short time convinced him that they increase gastric irritation, and the disposition to vomiting. Vomiting of blood, complete prostration, sudden death, and dangerous dysentery, were the effects of emetics, according to his observations. Even ipecacuanha, given with the greatest caution, was so dangerous, that it was preferable to abandon its use.

"In America, M. Bally prescribed, during the first two days, anodyne, mucilaginous, and laxative enemata: when the meteorism and tension of the epigastrium were considerable, he added camphor and quinine, in large doses, to combat prostration, and sometimes a considerable quantity of vinegar, to prevent decomposition. To prevent hypercatharsis, he prescribed laudanum, or the theriaca. Since his theory compelled him to resort to this disturbing treatment, he at least deserves credit for not administering them by the mouth.

"The warm bath, in which he kept the patient for several hours, and at different times, appeared to him a powerful auxiliary to the treatment, when there was no danger of pulmonary congestion. It would be more rational to fear a congestion of the head; a congestion which might be prevented by the application of ice to the cranium.

"If the warm bath is useful, it is not certain that the same remark may be made with regard to baths of bark and alcohol, which M. Bally did not employ, but which he recommended to the attention of practitioners. He did not employ the cold bath, which, it is said, is used by the negroes so successfully as to authorize a trial of it. I should not readily resort to such a measure in a disease which menaces both the head and chest. The case is not the same with regard to cold applications to the head: they are indicated whenever there is an afflux of blood to the head, and should be assisted by the abstraction of blood, and hot pediluvia. M. Bally recommends pediluvia, rendered stimulating by mustard and vinegar.

"Hot fomentations, applied to the epigastrium, epithems, with camphor, opium, and theriaca—frictions, with sulphuric or acetic ether, appeared to him to moderate the vomiting. Blisters (which he applied to the same part) are directly contra-indicated by the nature of the disease. Cups occasion intolerable and dangerous pain, if the epigastrium is sensible to pressure. The water of orange-leaves, of mint, ether and mint, should have been banished from the practice of a physician, who, in the multitude of post-mortem examinations which he made, almost always discovered a more or less marked state of phlogosis of the stomach. It doubtless was previously to his researches, that he prescribed liquid ammonia: after his investigations, he surely would have been on his guard against such a measure. Yet, when the alvine evacuations became excessive, he gave opiate mixtures, the root of columbo, cascarilla, catechu, and sulphuric acid, in union with the serpentaria. When meteorism of the abdomen was not a precursor of a critical movement,—when it was owing to extreme debility, or a gangrenous disposition,—(M. Bally does not say by what signs he recognised this 'debility'— this 'disposition,') he had recourse, not only to the exciting lavements already mentioned, but likewise to the internal use of the extract or tincture of bark, and also of ether and camphor. When there was hemorrhage, he resorted to cold, acidulated lotions: to the mineral lemonade; to the decoction of bark and serpentaria, acidulated; to the acetate of ammonia; to the sulphuric elixir of Minsicht; to the super-sulphate of alumine.

"M. Bally is certainly one of the physicians who have sacrificed least to a blind empiricism, and to the doctrines of Brown, in the treatment of yellow fever, and it is on this account that I have described his method rather than any other; because he persisted for a longer time in the employment of acidulous and emollient remedies. We now perceive that the yellow fever has been treated, in America, in the same manner as the typhus has been in Europe: consequently, the yellow fever being, in general, more fatal than the typhus, and the treatment being equally contra-indicated by the state of the organs in both countries, it is not surprising that the mortality from the one has been even more considerable, in America, than that of the other in Europe. It is proved by the researches of M. de Jonnes that, between the years 1796 and 1802, more than a quarter of the French troops sent to the Caribbe islands were cut off by the yellow fever. Whatever be the violence of this disease, such a result evidently demonstrates that the treatment hitherto employed should be abandoned. Certainly, it would be difficult to point out the impropriety of substituting another mode of treatment, or even of abandoning the disease to nature, in preference to continuing a practice so inefficient or injurious.

"'In the month of December, 1802,' says M. Bally, 'I was attacked by the prevailing disease, in consequence of sleeping on board a man-of-war, which was in the roadstead: here I was penetrated by a humid cold, from which I found it impossible to protect myself. The next day, I felt no indisposition; but on the following morning, at two o'clock, I was seized with a rigor, which lasted half an hour, and which was followed by considerable heat and profuse sweat; my body was immediately assailed throughout, with pains, and the kidneys, in particular, were violently affected. They persisted during five days, and that of the kidneys continued until the ninth; the fever was marked by a strong exacerbation towards evening, by intense heat,—more remarkable in the hands and feet,—and by an increase of the intense pain which pervaded the whole body. Sometimes I was sensible of some confusion of intellect; but I was not delirious. I preserved a state of uninterrupted calmness and tranquillity. My sleep was interrupted, and was seldom tranquil; my tongue was loaded, white in the centre, and clean on the edges: thirst moderate, salivation abundant, mouth clammy. The organs of taste and smell had acquired such acuteness, that I could distinguish, in water, the aromatic savor and odor communicated to it by the flowers which fell into the stream; a delicacy of perception to which I was a stranger during health. Whenever my feet were immersed in the water, I was seized with a general spasm, more sensibly and painfully felt in the stomach: the spasm was followed by pain and syncope; but after this first effect had passed, the pediluvium appeared to have a soothing effect, and I remained in it with pleasure. It was readily perceived that the stomach was the seat of an affection, from its liability to painful contraction, from the frequent eructations, vomiting, and want of appetite. A gentle purgative was administered, which was immediately rejected, and which, fortunately, produced no effect. Lavements occasioned rejections of whitish matters: the urine was free, and respiration easy. I could not support any kind of drink; every thing appeared to me either insipid and nauseous, or too strong: it was, therefore, necessary to confine myself to simple water. I remained in this state for ten days, and my convalescence was neither long nor painful. I took no kind of medicine. The effects of simple water were assisted by a general bath, by pediluvia, and by lavements.' "

Were I suffering under the yellow fever, I should certainly desire to be treated as M. Bally was; and I cannot but remark on the present occasion, the similarity of his conduct to that of Hildenbrand. Differing from Chirac, who employed the same method in his own case which he prescribed for his patients, these two physicians wisely preferred the danger of their disease to that of the treatment.

"There is one measure with regard to which experience has not yet pronounced; I mean the abstraction of blood. Almost all the physicians who have seen the yellow fever regret blood-letting in this disease. Some, Deveze and M. Dalmus among others, recommend it at the commencement, and when the symptoms have a very marked inflammatory character. A few, and among these Mosely, advise the repetition of blood-letting until the symptoms decrease in intensity. The first trials of this measure which M. Bally made, succeeded so badly that he hastened to follow an opposite plan. 'I observed,' he remarks, 'that the patients who were bled by the routine of practitioners of the country, died two days sooner than was usual in other cases; viz.: about the fifth, instead of the seventh day.' Independently of these results, we are not inclined to class venesection among the remedial measures in this disease, since it is seldom useful in gastro-enteritis. The only cases in which it can be resorted to with advantage is, when the lung is on the point of being inflamed, or delirium about to supervene."—Boisseau, page 342.

The preceding quotation will go to show how very cautious we should be in adopting active remedial agents in the treatment of a disease about which the faculty are so much divided.

Now that we have commented with some freedom on the opinions and practices of others, we solicit the same free and unbiassed examination of our own special and peculiar views, which we shall aim to unfold to our readers in as few words as possible.

Professor Leibig, in his admirable work on "Organic Chemistry," tells us that "The art of the physician consists in the knowledge of the means which enable him to exercise an influence on the duration of the disease; and in the removal of all disturbing causes, the action of which strengthens or increases that of the actual cause of disease."

"It is only by a just application of its principles that

any theory can produce really beneficial results. The very same method of cure may restore health in one individual which, if applied to another, may prove fatal in its effects. Thus, in certain inflammatory diseases, and in highly muscular subjects, the antiphlogistic treatment has a very high value; while in other cases blood-letting produces unfavorable results.

"The vivifying agency of the blood must ever continue to be the most important condition in the restoration of a disturbed equilibrium, which result is always dependent on the saving of time; and the blood must, therefore, be considered and constantly kept in view, as the most powerful cause of a lasting vital resistance, as well in the diseased as in the unaffected parts of the body."

"It is obvious, moreover, that in all diseases where the formation of contagious matter and of the exanthemata is accompanied by fever, two diseased conditions simultaneously exist, and two processes are simultaneously completed; and that the blood, as it were by reaction, (that is, fever,) becomes a means of cure, as being the carrier of that substance (oxygen) without the aid of which the diseased products cannot be rendered harmless, destroyed, or expelled from the body—a means of cure by which, in short, neutralization or equilibrium is effected."

We cannot but feel gratified in the perusal of Professor Loibig's very able, instructive and interesting treatise on animal chemistry, and finding that in no one particular do the researches of the learned Professor in the laws of animal life, or even the play of chemical affinities, so demonstrably unfolded by his labors, come in collision with our theory of life and of fever; we are led to feel more fully confirmed in the correctness of our views.

We have, in the preceding chapters, at some length laid before our readers at least the general principles on which all fevers should be treated. It here only remains for us to show, specifically, in what way we would apply those principles to practice in yellow fever. In this as in all other forms of fever, we recognize a variableness of type conformably to the modifying influence of the producing causes; hence, in some places and in some seasons it partakes more of the typhoid character than in others, at some times admitting a limited use of depletive remedies, while at other times it calls for the prompt and free use of tonics and of stimulants from the beginning.

Inasmuch as the forces of morbid action are more generally and more distressingly manifested in the stomach than in any other individual organ, it should claim our first attention. Should the irritation of this organ be great, with vomiting or retching to vomit, then we should first empty it by the administration of suitably warm diluent drinks, such as the teas of camomile, sage, or black snake root; so soon as the ordinary contents are thrown off, if the stomach does not then become settled or composed, we should proceed to allay its irritation by other means. This may be done by the application of mustard plasters to the pit of the stomach and to the extremities; while at the same time we administer a dose of laudanum, paregoric, essence of peppermint, aromatic spirit of hartshorn, or a draught of some grateful cordial of any kind that the patient may prefer.

The stomach being thus measurably composed, or suitable measures having been put in progress to achieve it, our next object should be to decide in our minds upon the propriety of abstracting blood; should the heat of the skin, the pain and sense of fulness of the head, the age, habits, and constitution of the patient, that is, being young, full habited and sound, indicate it, then should we take off just so much blood as would relieve the vascular system of any excess of tension that might exist, say, not more than about one pint of blood, thereby giving to the fluids more freedom and ease of circulation, while you leave on the solids a lighter burden to carry: ever bearing in mind that admirable caution of Professor Leibig, that the blood is the carrier of oxygen, the agent by and through which all restorations are accomplished.

Our next inquiry should be directed to the state of the bowels; if the circumstances of the case indicated the necessity of purging, such as fullness, pain, torpor or uneasiness, and whenever a spontaneous purging or looseness did not occur, then we should give from six to ten grains of calomel, with a half-grain or more (according to the irritability of the stomach,) of good denarcotised opium, or from fifteen to twenty drops of laudanum, and repeat every six hours if required, for two or three doses; and if it fails to act on the bowels in due time, say six or eight hours, then use the tincture of aloes and of senna, senna tea, cream of tartar, castor oil, or injections, until the desired effect is produced;—suffer the bowels thus to be gently but effectually evacuated, and when this has been thus accomplished, only aim afterwards to maintain a full natural action during the balance of the treatment, which can be done by the use of mild laxative pills, the saline purgatives, or the use of injections, as particular circumstances might indicate.

The stomach being composed, and the bowels having been put in motion, or evacuated, we should not wait for the full operation of the cathartic to be over, before we should proceed to administer one grain of quinine every hour, both by day and night, regardless of heat of skin or other symptoms of fever, such as a sense of fulness or pain of head or elsewhere. We are for losing no time in the administration of quinine in this disease, for the reason that its febrifuge and antiseptic virtues are called for more forcibly and earlier in this than in any other form of fever, to counteract the tendency to gangrene and mortification, which is threatening the whole system, particularly the stomach and bowels: as a suitable auxiliary to the febrifuge action of the quinine, we should allow our patients the limited use of any of the cool acidulated or alkaline drinks, such as weak lemonade, tamarind water, or solution of the citrate of potash, or the bicarbonates of potash or soda; or if circumstances indicated a preference to the vegetable diaphoretic teas, then use the infusion of the black snake-root, sage, camomile or other teas, either warm or cold.

During the continuance of the febrile symptoms, some one or other of these diaphoretic auxiliaries should be continued, and should the patient be at any time troubled with pain, delirium, or restlessness, then draw a blister over the back of the neck, or over the pit of the stomach. We have also found relief from the use of laudanum and camphire in doses of from three to five grains of camphire to six or eight drops of laudanum, to be repeated every five or six hours, as directed in the treatment of bilious fever, to be taken in lieu of, or in connexion with, some of the sweating teas. These sweating auxiliaries should be used only during the continuance of the strictly febrile symptoms, nor should they be used with such freedom as to run the patient into wasting sweats.

So soon as we shall have succeeded in bringing about a remission of febrile symptoms, we should then discontinue the use of the diaphoretics; but continue the regular use of the quinine, with the occasional use of camphire and opium.

Whenever we find our patients losing ground under this treatment, that is, that debility is still increasing—the disease assuming a still lower grade, under these circumstances, whether with or without febrile symptoms, we would do well to administer some of the most pleasant and acceptable of the diffusible stimulants, such as wine, milk-toddy, the malt liquors, panada, or such like, to be given every two or three hours, until some appreciable impression is made on the pulse, or an amelioration of symptoms in other respects occurred.

COUNTER-IRRITANTS.

In the onset of the disease, or during the first or second days of the attack, we should use mustard plasters to the stomach or extremities, with a view to relieve particular local distress, or to procure a revulsion from more vital internal structure of the body; but taking care at all times not to continue them on any spot long enough at a time to draw a blister. After the lapse of two or more days, should pain of the head, delirium, sickness of stomach or pain elsewhere still continue to distress the patient, in such cases we should seek relief by the drawing of a blister or blisters by the use of Spanish flies.

13

DIET.

Any light, wholesome, and easily digested food desired by the patient may be allowed. But inasmuch as the force of the disease is in a great measure spent upon the digestive organs, we should be particular both as to quantity and quality of the food indulged in.

For doses and modes of administering the several remedies recommended in this chapter, the reader will see chap. 16.

CHAPTER X.

OF INFLUENZA.

Influenza is that link in the chain of diseases which connects bad colds with continued fevers; its fever is generally of the typhoid character.

It appears for the most part as either an endemic or as an epidemic. It either assails the inhabitants of a country simultaneously, or spreads rapidly over a community.

It is generally of short duration, and not often a very serious disease.

Its prime causes are transitions of atmospheric temperature, and most probably connected with some peculiar derangement in its electric condition. Its visitations are most common in the fall, winter, or spring seasons.

In its attacks its symptoms are very much like those of a common cold, such as frequent sneezing, coughing, sense of fulness in the head, soreness of the breast, and sometimes a sense of stiffness and soreness of the whole muscular system. In some instances the attacks are so severe, or from some cause become so, that the patient has some of the usual symptoms of fever, such as chilly sensations, succeeded by flashes of heat, headach, hurried circulation, and so forth.

This disease is not usually dangerous, although there has sometimes been considerable mortality from it, especially among the aged and infirm.

TREATMENT.

When the attack is mild, which is most commonly the case, though the symptoms may continue for many days, all that is necessary is to avoid exposure, guard against the extremes of hot and cold, live temperately, and maintain the regular action of the skin, by bathing the feet in warm water at night, and making use of some warm sweating portions, such as pepper, ginger, or sage teas.

If a dry cough or difficult respiration attends, then make use of slippery elm, flax-seed, or other mucilaginous drink through the day, and take a dose of Dover's powder, paregoric, or laudanum, at night.

But if the attack should be violent, or from any cause the symptoms should become aggravated, with chilly sensations, alternated with flashes of heat, a hot, dry skin, with increased thirst, or headach, the disease then assumes a more serious aspect, or is of a lower grade; now, in addition to the warm bathing, the tea and the laudanum, a grain of quinine should be taken every two or three hours, until the patient is certainly mending. Children should use less corresponding to their ages.

There is sometimes such a similarity in the symptoms and character of influenza with that of mild typhus, that in some sections of country it has been given the name of winter fever, and if it is not precisely the same, it partakes much of the typhus character, and should be treated as such. See mild typhus, chap. 11.

Should the bowels become bound, open them by giving broken doses of salts, castor oil, or some mild purgative; but if they should be too laxative, restrain the looseness by giving six or eight drops of laudanum, or an equivalent of Dover's powders, or paregoric, one, two, three, or four times a day, as occasion may require, until the looseness is checked.

The diet should be light, though nourishing; consisting chiefly of liquids, of a nutritive character.

But this disease (as all others, from neglect, bad management, or otherwise) sometimes runs into a chronic form, and terminates in dropsy, or an enlargement and soreness of the spleen, or liver. If that should be the case, it will require the same treatment, as recommended in other cases of such chronic affections. See symptoms and treatment of such affections, chapter VI.

CHAPTER XI.

MILD TYPHUS, OR NERVOUS FEVER.

DESCRIPTION.—The only difference that can be discovered between mild typhus and common bilious fever, in the commencement of the disease, is, that the symptoms, in the commencement of the former disease, are slower in their progress, and it is longer before they arrive at a crisis: the disease also generally proves to be more protracted, if not more fatal; hence it has sometimes been called slow fever.

In the first presentation of any fever, physicians judge oftener of its character by the season of the year in which it appears, than from any thing else, unless there be some external appearance by which they can designate it; such as an eruption, or a change in the color of the skin, or some other equally marked symptom: or until the disease has run a time, and the appearances and symptoms have more fully developed themselves.

Such is the striking similitude in the features of mild typhus, and common bilious fever, in the onset of the disease, that we frequently hear physicians differing in opinion as to the real character of the fever, even when the subject is present before their eyes. This diversity of theoretical opinion would be a matter of little importance to the patient, provided they could understand and agree as to the best mode of meeting the indications of cure in his case: but when they are in the habit of drawing their prescriptions from books, and from names, and have modes of practice suited to the many titles given to fevers, then the case is different.

In other words, a recollection of what is contained in the printed pages of books, will profit the afflicted patient but little, provided the practitioner has not yet learned to read correctly the living pages of nature.

We consider it a matter of but little, or of secondary importance, to attempt to describe, and to make clear and well-marked distinctions in the character of fevers, with a view of explaining, or of pointing out their essential, or diagnostic features, since it is a matter of but little consequence, while, at the same time, it is a task of difficult accomplishment. He that holds out an idea that it can be done, is either deceived himself, or attempts to deceive others. It is impossible, in the nature of things, to be done; for the reason that fevers run into, and through each other, with such natural facility, that nothing short of the wisdom of deity could certainly and clearly analyse them. We have thought, from our experience and observation, that the truly enlightened physician might learn so to apply his modifying agents, in some cases, as to cause a fever to assume the many features at his will.

Yet still there are, for the most part, some marked differences, or characteristic symptoms. For example: the skin is not generally so hot and dry in the first stage of a mild typhus, as it is in the same stage of a bilious, or some other fevers, nor is the pulse, generally, so irritable and fretful; also, in well marked cases of typhus, there generally is more dejection of mind, torpor, and cloudiness of intellect: but even these symptoms are by no means uniformly distinct. In most other respects, the symptoms are precisely the same as in other fevers; varying in proportion to the combination of circumstances.

Although mild typhus and bilious fevers do occur in all seasons of the year, and in all climates, yet typhus is much more common in the winter and spring, and in cold climates, than bilious fever. Mild typhus is also as much a continued or remittent fever, as common bilious, or any other fever; generally abating in the after-part of the night, or fore-part of the day.

This link in the chain of fever, like all others, has been divided and sub-divided into several varieties; nearly as many as there are symptoms attending it. But we shall make only two divisions of it. This we shall call mild typhus, or the highest grade; since the attack is milder, the patient less prostrated, and its progress less rapid. The lower grade, and more malignant form, which runs its course much more rapidly, (even more rapidly than yellow fever,) we denominate cold plague, or spotted fever, and will be treated of in the next chapter.

CAUSES.

There have been many conjectures relative to the cause of this disease. Some have ascribed it to malaria; some to atmospheric transitions; others to contagion; while others, again, favor the opinion that it arises from animalculi, floating in the atmosphere. For our part, whenever we have seen it, we have been able to assign a combination of causes for it, and we are led to believe that its causes and their combinations are as various and as complicated as the circumstances of human existence.

SYMPTOMS.

There are generally several days of indisposition, or a premonitory state, giving us warning of its approach; such as lassitude, listlessness, slight, chilly sensations, alternated with flushes of heat, decline of appetite, weakness of the limbs—more or less of aching pains over the whole body. These symptoms gradually increase, until the ordinary signs of fever are developed; thirst becomes slightly increased, with increased heat on the surface of the body: sometimes sick stomach and vomiting, with considerable pain in the head and back.

Sometimes these symptoms are exceedingly mild, and the disease very slow in its progress. Individuals not unfrequently experience all the premonitory symptoms, and return again to health, without being confined; at other times they are more prompt and distressing, even as much, so as an attack of common bilious fever. In the first stage of this disease, and before the patient becomes weakened much, we have sometimes known the disease speedily terminated by the occurrence of a free and general perspiration, whether produced by nature or by art. The equilibrium is thus restored to the system, and the individual is restored again to health.

In confirmed cases, the symptoms generally become more aggravated as the disease progresses. The tongue, which in the beginning wore a white coat, now assumes a yellow-brown color; the natural secretions of the mouth and tongue are suspended, the tongue is dry, and a dark gummy matter adheres to the teeth and lips; a sense of dryness in the mouth and throat, or fauces, causes the patient to desire frequent small draughts of water, while his thirst in the true sense is not great. The skin undergoes frequent changes, being alternately too hot and too dry, then covered with a free and offensive perspiration, which quickly chills the skin, especially when exposed to the air. The brain, partaking of the general debility and perturbation, gives for the most part unsound manifestations; the patient either suffers from great restlessness, frequently running into delirium, a low indistinct muttering, or becomes stupid or comatose. In some cases the bowels are torpid, and the abdomen or belly becomes puffed or tympanitic.

In others, the patient is disposed to waste by too frequent evacuations from the bowels. In some instances, swelling of the throat or in the glands of the groins takes place. With the decline of strength twitchings of the muscles, more especially of the hands or feet, make their appearance, hickups come on, cold clammy sweats supervene, the pulse gradually declines, the extremities become cold, and death closes the scene.

The foregoing symptoms more or less attend the patient through the whole course of his protracted sufferings, which, under the common or usual treatment, is dragged out to ten, twenty, and, in many instances, to thirty days;

while, under what we conceive to be a more rational treatment, our experience has taught us that it can be brought to a salutary crisis in from five to ten days, or half the time.

TREATMENT.

To us the indications of cure seem to be, time, rest, suitably light nourishment, and the use of such mild and slightly modifying remedial agents as are best calculated to restore the lost tone, and impart a healthy balance, to the animal economy. In other words, in this more than in any other fever, do we stand opposed to that class of doctors who are ambitious of the title of bold, energetic practitioners; for the reason, that this is one of the conditions of the human system in which its vital energies are greatly diminished—one in which much mischief is frequently done by hyper-medication—a condition, in truth, in which less is to be apprehended from the disease than from the officious intermeddling of bold practitioners.

It has been our fate to witness the deeds of death, both from wanton depletion and from high and excessive stimulation.

OF BLOOD-LETTING.

We have seen a few, very few, cases, in which we have been satisfied that our patients were the better for a moderate bleeding. These cases were similar to those in which we recommend the use of the lancet in bilious fevers; they were young subjects, of full habit, laboring under a hurried respiration and circulation, with evident signs of increased determination and distressed condition of the head. In some such cases we have preferred taking blood from the temples, by cups or by leeches, to a general bleeding from the arm. But in the large majority of cases that have fallen under our care, we have taken no blood at all, and have found the simple occasional application of cold cloths sufficient to reduce the excess of heat, and to give at all times a partial relief to the pain of the head. But, as we have elsewhere remarked, cold applications should be cautiously made, and their effects carefully watched.

EMETICS.

As we have remarked in the treatment of bilious fever, so may we say here, that we have occasionally seen a prompt check put to symptoms of nervous fever by the early use of an emetic, especially when it was followed by the free use of some of the sweating teas, so as to produce the full sudorific effect. The indications for their use seem to us to be, the condition of the stomach and that of the head, at the time being.

For example, should the patient's stomach be oppressed with food or a flowing of bile into it, or should the distress of the head seem in any way referable to either condition of the stomach, then, we think, it would be best to commence our treatment by the use of an emetic of ipecacuanha. But if, on the other hand, there was irritability of stomach, or the stomach not suffering in any way with more or less of constipation or torpor of bowels, then we would prefer first using some gentle cathartic, such as a dose of calomel or blue mass, rhubarb, aloes, castor oil, senna, Epsom salts, or any other efficient and mild purgative that the patient may prefer.

Whenever the stomach and bowels have been once well evacuated of their common contents, we should thereafter only aim to keep up a regular natural action; and when the natural tone of the organ is not sufficient to accomplish this, then we should resort occasionally to the use of mild injections, or in some conditions to the use of mild laxative medicine.

So soon as we shall have relieved the stomach and bowels of any unnecessary or offending contents, then we would advise the patient to take one grain of quinine every two or three hours, using during the hot stage, or especially while the skin is hot and dry, as much pure cold water or water holding in solution a little super-carbonate of soda, or some of the sweating teas, taken either hot or cold, as the patient's appetite may crave, or as the powers of his stomach will enable him well to manage.

We are thus particular to recommend the use of fresh

cold water, (say about the temperature of common spring water,) for the reason that we know it to be one of nature's best and safest febrifuges, and for the additional reason, (strange as it may appear,) that we know that the common sense of mankind has not yet surmounted a prejudice to the contrary, that once was promulgated from the schools.

Whenever the skin relaxes under the use of the sweating remedies, then they should be suspended, or taken at longer intervals, so as to prevent any unnecessary wasting by excessive perspiration. The quinine portions, however, should be regularly continued, day and night, even to the period of crisis, or a general solution of diseased action.

We are not ignorant of the many high authorities that stand opposed to this practice, yet still our reason and experience both sustain us.

We know not how better to reconcile the conflicting opinions, than by supposing that those who have given to the world adverse experience, were either unfortunate in their selection of cases, or that they were excessive in the use of the remedies. We hold to the idea that there is such a thing as feeling one's way in the use of remedies, and in this form of fever perhaps more than any other, it can be safely done, for the reason that the symptoms are not urgent, the disease being so slow in its progress that it allows us time to wait, and to observe the effect of remedies.

Why then should we officiously hurry out of existence, one who in nature's hands alone, unaided, (except by good nursing,) would hold out fifteen, or twenty, or more days, and then even recover? In the course of the fever, particular symptoms are apt to occur, calling for some special attentions, such as the existence of pain, sick stomach, or vomiting. These symptoms should be relieved by the use of essence of peppermint, paregoric, or laudanum, or the effervescing draught; or the coming on of bowel complaint in some form or other: when these symptoms assume the dysenteric form, that is, where there is pain and straining, a frequent inclination to stool, while at the same time there is a retention of fœcal matter, then have the bowels gently evacuated by small doses of salts or oil, then allay the intestinal irritation by the use of Dover's powders, paregoric, or laudanum, and warm fomentations or mustard plasters to the abdomen. But when the disease assumes the form of looseness or wasting discharges, then we should cautiously restrain such action by the use of mild astringents or opiates, such as paregoric, Dover's powders, or laudanum, repeated as circumstances might require.

DELIRIUM.

Whenever delirium supervenes, we should endeavor to calm the irritation of the brain by the use of camphor and laudanum, from three to five grains of camphor to about a quarter of a grain of opium, or six or eight drops of laudanum, to be repeated every four or six hours, and when obstinate, draw a blister on the back of the neck.

The use of camphor and opium, or laudanum, we have not confined to cases in which a delirium exists: we have found great benefit from their use whenever the patient seems to be losing ground, or sinking to a dangerously low grade.

Whenever the prostration of the patient becomes marked, (we should not wait as has been the practice of some, for signs of actual sinking,) he should be sustained by the guarded use of some of the diffusible stimuli, such as whiskey, wine, milk-toddy, wine-whey, the malt liquors, or such like, giving the patient always the choice of his drink. When the distilled liquors are used, we have usually recommended about a table spoonful once in three or four hours, or other things in the same ratio.

The occurrence of muscular twitchings (what is called by the learned subsultus tendinum) or of hiccups, will require no special treatment, inasmuch as they are merely signs of the state of the patient, and the tendency of the case. For remedies and doses of remedies recommended in this chapter, the reader will see chap. 16.

TYPHUS GRAVIOR.

By this term we understand nothing more than an aggravated form, or grade of typhoid fever, aggravated by the particular causes or circumstances of its existence. It is in reality the same disease that has been called putrid fever, plague, spotted or petechial, pestilential, malignant, camp, or jail fever, only taking different names from the circumstances of its origin.

It would be an unnecessary waste of our own and of the reader's time, to go into a detail of the special causes, or the particular treatment of this grade of fever, since by referring to what has been said of typhus mitior, or mild typhus, he will readily understand that of the gravior. It is to be treated upon the same general principles, only being more vigilant to watch its progress, and be more liberal in the use of the counteracting or remedial agents. That is to say, we should use quinine, and the stimulating diaphoretics more freely, and introduce the use of the diffusible stimulants more promptly. Since the symptoms, treatment, attentions in nursing and diet, in all very low and protracted cases of all fevers, are very much if not identically the same; and we have been more explicit in these particulars in the chapter on bilious fever than elsewhere. We refer the reader to that chapter for further instructions.

CHAPTER XII.

COLD PLAGUE, OR SPOTTED FEVER.

DESCRIPTION.

This is a low grade and malignant fever of the typhoid type: we consider it in many respects to be a different disease from the typhus gravior of other countries, while still in some of its features it bears a striking resemblance.

This formidable disease first made its appearance in New England in 1806. About the year 1810 or '12, it became so general in the northern and eastern portion of the United States as to be recognised as an epidemic; from thence it gradually spread south and west, until in the course of a few years it had traversed the whole union; leaving traces of its destructive powers wherever it went.

It was our fortune to witness its movements and its fatal ravages on several different theatres. In the city of Philadelphia we had our first introduction to it; in the city of Baltimore we witnessed something more of it; in the state of Virginia we have both seen and felt its influence; and in the state of Tennessee we still witnessed more of it. In the different places where we met with the disease, we have occupied the stations both of spectators and actors; we have heard the words of wisdom falling from the lips of the medical philosophers and advisers, while at the same time our eyes have been cast with deep interest on the living pages of suffering humanity.

CAUSES.

This disease happening to make its appearance during the time of the late war with Great Britain, and at a time when the United States soldiers were passing to and fro through the different portions of the Union, induced the belief with many that the disease had originated in the camps, and that it was propagated by contagion.

We regret that the character of our present enterprise, (being one of simple practical utility,) prohibits us from indulging in any speculations on this subject. We indulge the hope, however, that at some future day, and on some other occasion, it may be thought fit to speak, not only on the laws that regulated this epidemic, but of the laws of he movements of other epidemics; we shall for the present content ourselves with remarking that in all probability some peculiar condition of the atmosphere attended the disease whenever and wherever it appeared.

Since the period at which this disease first made its appearance in the epidemic form, the same or a similar disease has again and again, either in an endemic or sporadic manner, presented itself in different parts of this union.

It is most common in cold countries, and in the colder seasons of the year; it has hence frequently received the name of winter fever, as well as that of winter typhus.

SYMPTOMS.

In severe attacks of cold plague, the patient is suddenly stricken down, with violent pains in the limbs, body, or, more commonly, in the head; indeed, there is no particular location for the pain, it may be any where; we have known it to be the nose, the cheek, the knee, the side, or elsewhere. This local or general distress (as the case may be) is attended with an increased coldness over the whole surface of the body, with such diminished sensibility, that a reaction is not or cannot be readily restored; and the patient's existence is thus oftentimes terminated in the course of four or five hours.

The appearance of the tongue undergoes little or no change except that it is pale and the breath colder than usual, the pulse generally quicker and weaker than in any other grade of fever; it is sometimes even imperceptible at the wrists. Such are the ordinary and most striking symptoms. It is called spotted fever, when purplish blotches or spots make their appearance on the surface of the body.

Such spots are indicative of gangrene, or at least of a tendency to gangrene or mortification.

The tongue, in such conditions, assumes a dark hue, and dark-colored discharges are apt to take place from the stomach and bowels, somewhat like that of yellow fever.

TREATMENT.

The indications of cure are, first, to produce reaction, and, secondly, to maintain and to rightly regulate the reaction when produced. In the attacks of this disease, the system, both internally and externally, or, in the language of the physiologists, both the internal and external surfaces of relation, are in a state of inactivity, or of torpor, as is evinced by the coldness of the skin, depression of arterial action, and diminished sensibility to the impressions of stimuli of any kind. This state of things points to us, in language too clear and too strong to be misunderstood, the propriety, yea, the absolute necessity, of arousing the system from such alarming and such death-like prostration. For the accomplishment of this object, we know no better means, no steps more rational, than to restore the lost animal heat by artificial means, such as warm rooms, warm clothing, heated substances; such as bricks, bags of salt or sand, applied about the body of the patient; stimulating the external surface with mustard plasters, and the frequent use of internal stimuli; hot toddy, wine, cordials, spirit of hartshorn, red pepper tea, small doses of laudanum, and such like articles.

So soon as signs of reaction begin to manifest themselves, our next care should be to see that we do not overact the case, and destroy the feeble energies of life by excessive stimulation; for our object should be to bring back all of the organs of the system to the healthy performance of the natural functional duties, and no more: and, when thus restored, endeavor to maintain the healthy balance by means of the appropriate stimuli to each and to every organ, and thus to guard against the danger of a relapse. For this purpose, we know of no article so appropriate as the sulphate of quinine, taken in doses of one grain every two or three hours. If, indeed, as it sometimes happens after the reaction has been fully established, and, after the lapse of some days, signs of local inflammation, or congestion, should exist in any part of the body, under such circumstances, we should seek relief by the use of cups or blisters; for we rarely, if ever, have found it necessary to abstract blood from the arm. We, however, are not ignorant of the fact, that practices and opinions opposed to us, in this particular, have been pursued and promulgated from some of the high places of the medical profession. Let us, for example, here cite one such.—See Medical Statistics of the United States Army, published in 1840; page 267. Surgeon Lawson says:

"By far the most fatal disease of Louisiana, however, whether in our city or the low lands of the country, is the congestive form of fever, or, as it is here called, the cold plague. It is an insidious enemy, attacking, most commonly, the weak and enfeebled, and those laboring under mental depression. In many instances, the subject of the disease, before he himself or those around him are aware of it, becomes cold in the extremities, and on the superficies of the body generally; with the exception, perhaps, of the region of the chest, the blood retreats to the interior of the system, and the patient is at once prostrated. The vital organs being overwhelmed, the system cannot, of itself, react; and not unfrequently, all the means of art are of no avail in removing the load of oppression. There are other instances, however, in which the disease, although always insidious, and never without danger, is less severe in its attacks. In these cases the system may, with a little assistance, react efficiently, (it seldom, of itself, makes a successful effort,) and, after a protracted struggle, prevail over the disease.

"Under the first form of the disease, the primary indication seems to be, to restore the circulation to the extremities, by the application of hot water to the feet and legs, and blisters and sinapisms to the extremities and other parts of the body; by constant and long-continued frictions with stimulating substances; and by repeated doses of the diffusible stimuli.

"Having restored the circulation to the extreme vessels, and heat to the surface, our next object will be to relieve the engorged organs by repeated small bleedings, consecutively increased. These efforts, aided by the operation of one or more cathartics, will place the patient in a fair way for recovery; when subsequent treatment will depend altogether upon existing circumstances. In the second modification of the disease, blood must be taken away immediately, and its abstraction continued until the congestion is relieved.

"Calomel, as a purgative, may at once be given and repeated (perhaps even twice) with advantage.

"This terrible disease invaded our damp, crowded, and ill-ventilated prison-room, and instantly struck down two or three of its inmates. One of these, who was attacked after one o'clock, was found, in the morning, motionless, pulseless, and senseless; nay, he scarcely breathed. He was immediately put in hot water up to the knees, and was well rubbed over the body with warm salt, and other stimulating substances, whilst diffusible stimuli were freely administered; but it was all to no purpose. In spite of every effort to resuscitate him, he quickly succumbed. He once, for a moment, opened his eyes, and nodded assent to something that was said or done to him; but as I was preparing to bleed him, he relapsed into a state of insensibility, and passed away without another sign of life. In another case, the circumstances of the attack were similar, but less severe. In this instance, the system reacted in some measure; but it was a feeble effort, and the patient expired in the struggle."

With the preceding description, by Surgeon Lawson, with the facts stated, and even with the indications of cure pointed out by him, we are pleased to say that we entirely concur; but when we come to the application of means to meet those indications, we are compelled to differ: we do not, either, oppose the general means used; but we must object to the use of the lancet under such circumstances as have just been cited. In the one case, "while he was preparing to bleed his patient, he relapsed, and died." In the other, he tells us "that the system reacted in some measure." In this case, we have a right to infer that he did bleed: but, unfortunately, that patient, too, expired.

From what mode of reasoning, either on the laws of life, or on the laws of disease, he could feel justified in taking blood in either of the cases cited, we are utterly at a loss to divine.

We know that a vulgar prejudice still exists in the minds of some people, that we should open a vein to resuscitate from a fit of fainting, whether produced from moral or physical causes. Some men may even think it right to draw blood to recover persons from the sedative effects of a continued exposure to extreme cold, the mere abstraction of animal heat. But to our feeble and humble intellects, the sense of such a practice has never yet been made manifest. The spilling of blood in all such cases to us has seemed like unto that of the bloodshed of war; more frequently the offspring of error than of wisdom.

Surgeon Lawson is also an advocate for the prompt use of calomel. So soon as a reaction is fully established, should circumstances indicate the necessity of evacuating the stomach and bowels, then we have no objection to its prudent use, being careful, however, not to add to the patient's debility by too many or too plentiful discharges.

It may even be possible that the presence of a dose of calomel in the stomach or bowels, by its local irritation, might aid in producing a reaction; but we should see that its cathartic effects did not counteract its salutary virtues. With this view of the subject, we would prefer, at least during the period of depression, to use stimulating injections, and to endeavor so to qualify the matter of injection as to obtain a purely stimulant effect, or a stimulant and cathartic effect, as particular circumstances might indicate.

Whenever the patient shall have been successfully conducted through the cold stage into the fully developed state of reaction, our next object should be to conduct him through the febrile condition, when such condition exists, by as short and as safe a process as possible. We have already given a brief outline of the principles on which we should proceed. It now only remains for us to make some comments on the treatment of particular symptoms, and in particular cases. We wish the reader to know that this disease, when it runs into a febrile state, may, like other fevers, be attended with local congestion and even inflammations (such, however, is not often the case). Whenever and wherever such symptoms do occur, they should be treated as recommended in the other forms of fever already described; for example, if there be much pain in the head or delirium, then have blisters drawn on the back of the neck, and allay the pain and irritation of the brain or its membranes by the administration of doses of camphor and laudanum, in the proportion of from three to five grains of the former, with from six to eight drops of

the latter, and relieve the febrile heat by the use of some
the diaphoretic teas; and in case of a want of due action from the bowels, then have them cautiously moved by a dose of calomel, or the use of mild injections. But should the pain, be located on the side, throat, stomach, bowels, or elsewhere, then apply to the distressed parts mustard plasters, or plasters of Spanish flies, and let your general treatment in all other respects be such as just described.

It not unfrequently happens that this disease runs into the form of mild typhus fever. In such cases, the author has found the best results to follow the use of quinine, in grain doses, as before described for that form of fever.

In some cases it is difficult to maintain the natural animal temperature in the extremities; in such cases, mustard or blister plasters should be applied to the wrists and ankles.

When purplish spots make their appearance under the skin, (what the medical writers call petechia,) this symptom should be considered as a sign of, or as a tendency to, gangrene or mortification; the tongue now asumes a darker hue, and dark discharges are apt to take place from the stomach and bowels; when such symptoms occur, they call for the immediate free use of quinine, one grain every hour or two, day and night, with a more or less free use of some diffusible stimuli; such as wine-whey, milk or other toddy, the malt liquors, with the occasional use of opiates or laudanum in some form or other, to procure rest or ease; and blister plasters to be applied wherever particular local distress may indicate.

During the whole course of the treatment, the patient should be indulged in such light and wholesome diet, as he may desire, and as his stomach is capable of digesting.

CHAPTER XIII.

SCARLET FEVER.

DESCRIPTION.

This disease has derived its name from the scarlet color of the skin under fever, or the eruption of the fever. The fever which attends it may be of any grade, from the highest to the lowest. The disease may also vary in degrees of virulence or malignity, from the slightest irritation of the skin to that of the plague. It occurs at all seasons of the year, but is most common in the fall, winter, and spring months. It assails most generally the young, is most fatal with children, while the matured and aged are by no means exempted from it. It sometimes appears as an epidemic disease, spreading over extended regions of country; but most commonly it appears as an endemic in particular towns, villages, and country situations. Whenever it assumes an epidemic character, it is apt to appear with great malignity, spreading alarm and death wherever it goes. It has been divided into a variety of kinds or species, acording to particular symptoms attendant on its march.

By some writers it has been confounded with putrid sore throat, while with others it has been viewed as a distinct disease.

For our part, we can readily conceive the general type of disease to run into many forms, or for two or more forms or symptoms to be blended together, so as to make up the catalogue of names under which it has been described by the different writers;—such as scarlatina anginosa, scarlatina metis, scarlatina maligna, cynanche maligna, &c. We shall simply aim to hold up the disease in its most general and striking characteristic features, and in that way which we shall consider to be the most important in a practical point of view.

CAUSES.

Of the prime causes and of the prime specific element or elements that give rise to this disease, we can say but little.

Its origin ever has and probably ever will continue to be a subject of unfathomed inquiry; whether it is generated by atmospheric changes, or from organic changes in the human body, wrought by other causes, we know not. Nearly all writers concur, however, in the belief that the disease, when produced, may be propagated by contagion, that is, by the effluvia emanating from the bodies of the sick. One strong argument in favor of its contagious nature and specific character is, that persons seldom have it more than once in their lives. In this respect it obeys the laws of the other eruptive diseases, about the contagious nature of which there is less dispute, to wit: smallpox and measles.

SYMPTOMS.

This disease is sometimes very insidious in its approach: children who have made no complaint in the forenoon, but are seen to take, as usual, interest in their toys, have been frequently known to die before night. Such patients make little or no complaint; some slight chilly sensations pass over them; perhaps they will make some mention of pain of head, or soreness of the throat, or of sickness of stomach. On indisposition, we find the tongue coated with a moist white fur, through which the red papillæ are seen peeping over its whole surface, some faint spots at the same time may be seen in the roof and palate of the mouth; the extremities and even the whole body feels too cold; the breath even is colder than natural, the circulation is languid, the pulse feeble, indeed, all the signs of life seem gradually to fade away, and the laws of death triumph over those of life seemingly without a struggle; as though one were dying from the mere abstraction of animal heat.

In other instances the attack comes on suddenly, with violent pukings, or with both puking and purging—

bearing a striking resemblance to the first stage of the Asiatic cholera. But so soon as the evacuations are checked, which is usually done under the influence of external and internal stimuli of some kind, then it is that the florid eruption, or the peculiar soreness of the throat, or both, proclaim in language not to be mistaken, the true nature of the disease.

Again: We sometimes see the disease coming on like an attack of any other fever, with chill, followed by increased heat of skin, and other conditions usually attendant on fevers.

The eruptions or petechial spots usually make their appearance within the first forty-eight hours from the attack. We sometimes witness cases in which the petechial spots are well developed, without any soreness of the throat at all; while in other cases, we see the soreness of the throat without the eruption. The eruption is first visible in the roof of the mouth, next it appears on the external surfaces, earliest about the neck and chest, or those parts of the body usually the warmest and best protected by clothing. After a continuance of some three or four days, the spots gradually fade away in very slight cases, without any shedding of the cuticle, or the external coat of the skin. But in those cases where the eruption is more fully developed, the desquamation or shedding of the skin becomes more considerable.

Scarlet fever may be distinguished from the measles by the more florid color of the eruption, and by its being more diffused, the spots less elevated and less distinct than in measles, although the eruption in either disease may become confluent. In scarlatina, cough is a rare attendant; while in measles it is an invariable symptom.

TREATMENT.

The indications of cure are, to watch over the symptoms of each individual case, to keep the disease in its natural channel, and endeavor to conduct the patient in safety through the different metamorphoses or changes necessarily attendant on its march.

Let us now illustrate: Should a case set in with symptoms of prostration, or that fading away, as intimated in our first view of the subject, then we should endeavor to bring about as prompt a reaction, return of natural warmth, and developement of febrile symptoms, as we can; for this purpose we should restore the animal heat by external heat, applied in the form of warm water to the feet and legs, warm bricks, bags of heated sand or salt, mustard to the extremities, and the prompt and reasonable use of warm diffusible stimuli, taken inwardly, such as hot toddy, or the more permanent stimuli of ginger or pepper tea. So soon as a reaction is thus brought about, or, if during the reaction, circumstances indicate a fullness or oppression of the stomach, then we may seek to relieve that organ by the administration of warm diluents, or warm salt water, or a little ipecacuanha added to the salt water if necessary to excite vomiting. The salt emetic, or the salt water with the ipecacuanha, seems to have produced a better effect than other emetics in such cases, by virtue of its combining an antiseptic, a tonic, or a condiment property, to that of its mere evacuating effect. But we think it more than probable, reasoning both from analogy and from experience, that a grain of quinine taken either alone or in combination with some diffusible stimulus, every hour or two, will be found preferable in such cases to any other practice.

The indications in the second view of the disease would seem to be, to let the stomach and bowels first rid themselves of their ordinary or offending contents, then to restrain their action by the use of mustard plasters to the stomach, while laudanum and peppermint are taken internally, in such doses and at such intervals as may be necessary to accomplish the desired object.

So soon as the stomach and bowels have become quieted, and the natural reaction established, then proceed to treat the case upon general principles, as in a case setting in with any other symptoms.

Cases occurring as represented under the third view of symptoms, should be treated by the mere use of some warm diluent drinks or slightly diaphoretic teas, so as to maintain a regular and natural developement of the disease. Should the eruption or the determination to the skin seem too faint, with signs of distress on any of the internal surfaces of relation, then should the patient take a grain of quinine occasionally, say once in two or three hours, with a view of sustaining a natural and a safe progression of symptoms, or metamorphoses; that is, the progressive transformation of symptoms, or the full development and elimination of the disease, by and through the skin.

In all cases, however violent, the forming stage of the disease may be so soon as we shall see the eruption or the petechial spots sufficiently manifest on the skin; our remaining object should be, to conduct the case safely to its natural crisis.

To accomplish this task, after attending to the particular symptoms just pointed out, the treatment will consist in giving one grain of quinine every two or three hours, regularly by day and by night, for the purpose of maintaining the natural play of organic action. When the heat and dryness of the skin are too great, then we should administer some of the diaphoretic teas, to aid the quinine in its operation on the depurative organs—such as sage, pepper, or snake-root teas; and whenever the grade of fever becomes very low, and the debility great, in such cases we should substitute some of the diffusible stimuli in lieu of the diaphoretic teas—such as wine whey, toddy, panada, &c., once in every three or four hours.

Should the tension of the vascular system, together with the signs of local inflammation, or of congestion, clearly call for it, then blood should be taken from the arm, according to the principles of restriction heretofore pointed out.

The practitioner should never lose sight of the fact, that this disease, like most other febrile affections, is variable in its type, and that our practice should always correspond to the variableness of the type and circumstances of particular cases.

In regard to the local distress about the parotid gland,

or the internal structure of the throat, we have only to say, that we consider this as one of the attendant phenomena of the disease, and that as a symptom it requires not much special attention—for that which relieves the system of the febrile affection relieves its local features.

We, however, admit the propriety of using astringent gargles of oak tea, sage tea, and alum, internally, while we apply soothing liniments, such as camphorated liniments, opodeldoc, and such like, externally. Of the efficacy of blisters to the part we have some doubts; leeches may avail something in lessening the inflammation, while cupping would be too irritating to be borne by the patient. Whenever a tendency to suppuration is marked, we may lessen the patient's suffering by applications of slippery elm or flax-seed poultices to the parts; and so soon as matter is well formed, proceed to let it out by a puncture with a lancet.

CATHARTICS.

The use of cathartic remedies we consider as contraindicated in this, as well as in all other eruptive or exanthematous diseases, excepting to a very limited degree, and under particular circumstances; for the reason, that they have a tendency to suppress, or to throw the diseased manifestations on the internal surfaces, or on internal tissues more highly vitalized and more immediately connected with, and essential to, life: thus inverting the natural order of the animal economy, which is to direct the morbific matter, whatever it be, to be cast off by the skin.

With this view of the subject, we are led to pursue that course which leaves or maintains the stomach and bowels, if not in a quiescent, at least as near to a natural condition as we can. If too much torpor exists, then use mild injections, or mild cathartics, such as senna and Epsom salts, castor oil, or rhubarb.

Since scarlatina is most common to youth, and to children at that period of life when worms are most common, we have in many cases found the presence of worms to be a considerable impediment to the natural, and we might say, healthy progress of the disease, experience has taught us the propriety of inquiring into and attending to the removal of worms, whenever their presence is suspected from the age or other conditions of the patient.

We have been led to recommend the prompt and free use of vermifuges at an early period of the disease, whenever we suspected the existence of worms; for this purpose we would recommend the use of the wormseed oil, or the spirit of turpentine, giving preference to these vermifuges in scarlatina for the reason, that while they were effectual worm medicines, they disturbed not the regular progress of the eruption or the fever.

DIET.

During the progress of the symptoms patients would do well to confine themselves principally to a light, warm, and fluid diet, such as tea, coffee, soup, panada, scald milk, and such like. For remedies, and their doses, see chap. 16.

CHAPTER XIV.

MEASLES, [RUBEOLA.]

DESCRIPTION.—Measles is a contagious disease, characterized by a peculiar eruption attended with fever; its first stage resembling very much the commencement of a cold: heaviness of the head, coughing, and sneezing. It appears epidemically, and is also propagated by infection. It is most common during the winter and spring seasons. Children are most prone to its attacks, while the aged are not exempted from it. Persons who have been once brought under its influence are seldom liable to a second attack.

CAUSES.

Of the prime causes of measles we are just as ignorant as we are of the prime causes of scarlatina. Like smallpox, it has been ascribed to the crowded condition of families in cities and villages; the consequent want of purity or the vitiation of atmosphere, and the want of personal cleanliness.

SYMPTOMS.

The attack is usually announced by a general uneasiness; chilliness; shivering; more or less pain of head and limbs; sometimes sick stomach and vomiting; a heaviness and fulness about the eyes; tumefaction of the face; frequent sneezing, with a flow of tears from the eyes and nose; a dry cough, with some soreness of the throat. With the progress of these symptoms, come the usual signs of fever: a hot and dry skin, augmented thirst, increased arterial action, and hurried respiration. The tongue now begins to put on a white coat. To these symptoms, after a lapse of three, four, or sometimes five days, succeed eruptions on the skin; first, about the face, neck, and chest, then over the whole surface of the body. The disease may frequently be recognized by the peculiar redness of the eyes, and the eruption on the roof and palate of the mouth, before it has made its appearance on the exterior surfaces of the body. The eruption usually commences in distinct spots, like flea-bites, but they sometimes run together, so as to give to the face and neck one uniform red appearance. The eruption differs from that of scarlatina, in producing a roughness or elevation of the surface, not common to scarlatina; the weeping of the eyes, and intolerance of light, is also a symptom that does not belong to scarlet fever. This eruption continues from four to six days, attended with more or less of a febrile condition; then subsides, with a shedding of the cuticle, or outer coat of the skin, in bran-like scales. The casting off of the cuticle usually commences on the fourth day, and becomes general on the sixth day; by which time all signs of fever commonly disappear.

The time that intervenes between the first impression, or exposure to the contagion, and the actual commencement of the disease, varies from a few days to two or three weeks; but from seven to nine days may be considered as the ordinary course of experience.

Some more or less of febrile action, from the beginning to the period of desquamation, seems necessary to accomplish the objects of the animal economy. The tongue is covered with a white coat; the appetite fails; the taste is perverted; the pulse usually full, frequent and soft: patient restless. Remissions of fever commonly take place every morning, while the symptoms become again aggravated during the evenings. In this respect, the fever obeys the common laws of other febrile affections.

When measles occur in healthy subjects, under favorable circumstances of weather and of attention, it is usually a mild and manageable disease; but when under other circumstances,—circumstances calculated to interrupt the regular development of the disease, and complete restoration,—then comes the danger. In other words, we have less to fear from the disease than from its consequences; or the consequences resulting from any interruption of its natural progression, and completion of its course of symptoms.

TREATMENT.

The indications of cure are to conduct the patients, as in other eruptive diseases, through the regular and natural stages and changes, inherent in the nature of the disease. To accomplish this, in most cases, requires no particular remedial aids.—The most important thing to be observed is, to preserve a uniform and suitable temperature: see that the system receives no shock from the transitions of temperature; either by passing from a higher to a lower, or from a lower to a higher temperature. Let the clothing be suited to the weather, and the patient's room be kept comfortably warm and dry; while, at the same time, it is furnished with a sufficiency of pure and fresh air. The diet should be light, easily digested, and mostly fluid. It is only when the symptoms begin to vary from their natural course, that remedial agents should be brought into use.

The practice of officiously intermeddling, under promises of cure, has generally done more harm than good. It is nature's laws that effect all the cures: the doctor should be her servant, interpret her laws, consult her will, remove obstacles, and offer facilities to achieve her will. If eruptive diseases have a prescribed course to run, and a given time to accomplish that course, as all enlightened observers know to be the natural law, and the patient is doing well in nature's hands, why, then, should we officiously intermeddle?

Whenever an individual is discovered to be coming under the influence of the measles, our first object should be to see that he is placed under favorable circumstances for the disease to run its course without any interruption from external causes; and the next care should be to have the characteristic features of the disease fully evolved. If the tone and energy of the individual are not such as to bring out the eruption in due time, then the operations of nature should be assisted by bathing the feet and legs in warm water, and administering, internally, at the same time, some warm and slightly stimulating teas; such as sage, red pepper, ginger, black snake-root teas, or, in obstinate cases, wine-whey, mint-julep, hot toddy, spirit of hartshorn: or that which is still preferable to the above, will be to give a grain of quinine once in two or three hours. The eruption being thus evolved, our next care should be to maintain it in its regular and natural course, without running to any excess.

The practitioner should bear in mind the well-settled truth, that the fever of measles is subject to the same variableness of type that is common to other fevers; that is, that it may be of a high or of a low grade—it may be very slight, or it may be the reverse. True it is, that some writers of limited experience, of limited range of inquiry and of thought, have assumed the position that the type of fever is always inflammatory, and that, consequently, depletive remedies of some kind or other are always more or less indicated. It would be departing from the spirit of this treatise to enter into an argument on this subject: enough, we hope, has been already said, in our theory of fever, to lead the reader's mind to correct conclusions. These remarks are intended to direct the attention of the practitioner to the necessity and propriety of accurately discriminating and weighing the symptoms and circumstances of the case, that he may decide on the propriety of abstracting blood. Whenever the disease occurs in young and plethoric subjects, attended with high grade of action, and more especially where it is attended with much local distress, such as pain of the head, distress of throat or lungs, with tense pulse and hurried arterial action, then should the patient lose a moderate portion of blood; such a quantity as would take off the excess of tension, and thereby lessen the danger of local inflammation, or of congestion: never forgetting that some fever is necessary, and that the blood is the medium through which the restorations are to be achieved.

EMETICS.

There is no one of the depletive measures used in the treatment of measles in which there is a more general concurrence of opinion than in that of the use of emetics.

This class of remedies is indicated when there is difficulty of breathing, from an accumulation of mucus in the windpipe or lungs, in cases of much soreness of throat, and indeed in many cases, to promote the developement of the eruption.

In all of these conditions they afford relief by the immediate evacuations in part, but mainly by the prompt revulsions or determination to the external surfaces, which effect should always be promoted by the aid of some warm stimulating diaphoretic teas, such as sage, red pepper, snakeroot, and so forth. As an emetic in such cases we have used the ipecacuanha, either in substance or in the form of its vinous tincture. The lobelia has also been recommended in similar conditions.

CATHARTICS.

We have already said that cathartics, as curative agents, are seldom indicated in eruptive fevers; we should only aim to relieve the intestinal canal of any excess of fulness, and afterwards to maintain a natural, regular and healthy action. For this purpose the practitioner should use the mildest laxatives, or mild injections, whenever the condition of the patient would call for it. It is better to evacuate the bowels in the early stage of the disease, for the reason, that if you make a sensible impression on the bowels at or about the period of desquamation, there is danger of running the patient into a troublesome bowel complaint.

If, on the contrary, from any cause, an unnatural or excessive action of the bowels should occur, in such cases they should be relieved by the judicious use of simple astringents, or of opiates, or a combination of the two classes of remedies. Generally we find that the compound spirit of lavender, or a dose or two of paregoric, or a few drops of laudanum taken in an effusion of some of the vegetable astringents, such as tho root of the blackberry or the inner bark of some of the oaks, will answer every purpose.

Whenever the symptoms are not such as to call for the depletive aid of the lancet, cathartics or emetics, and still the febrile heat and restlessness are amounting to distress, in such cases we should seek relief by gently exciting the action of the skin, by the administration of some of the diaphoretic teas, or of the alkaline diaphoretics, such as the bicarbonate of potash or of soda, or by the soothing effects of small doses of paregoric or laudanum.

In some instances we find the measles attended with a low grade or typhoid type of fever, even from the commencement; such are rare occurrences, and are to be met with only where persons are much crowded, and other unfavorable circumstances for health; in all such cases we would advise the use of quinine in grain doses, once in every two or three hours; and should the signs of great depression and prostration supervene, we would, under such circumstances, add the guarded use of some diffusible stimulus to that of quinine.

Patients recovering from measles should ever be extremely cautious of exposure to sudden transitions of temperature, or to any imprudence in diet, since one of the critical periods of the disease is that at which the desqua mation takes place or the fever subsides. Improper exposure to a cold and damp atmosphere is apt to result in some troublesome affection of the lungs, bowels or elsewhere; so also improper indulgence in food may bring on a troublesome disease of the bowels. Patients should continue to be guarded against any of the above indicated errors, for many days, even until their usual strength is restored.

CHAPTER XV.

PUERPERAL OR CHILD-BED FEVER.

This is a disease peculiar to women after delivery. It has been thought to be sometimes epidemic; and many respectable physicians have believed it to be propagated by contagion.

CAUSES.

This fever is most probably a consequence of lesions, or other mechanic injuries received by the womb and its appendages, including all the structure involved in the act of parturition or childbearing, so as to prevent them from performing their natural and proper functions; we mean here not those duties which belong to their action in health, but the performance of those duties, viz., the depurative functions by which the organs are again brought back to their former healthy condition. To these fixed and definable causes should be added that of the diminished general tone of both body and mind—a necessary consequence of the physical labor, pain, and mental anxiety, inseparably connected with the parturient process.

The external causes are, a cold and damp atmosphere, uncomfortable circumstances of existence, external causes of mental depression or perturbation.

SYMPTOMS.

The attack of the rigor or chill of a true puerperal fever, usually comes on after a lapse of more than forty-eight hours—that is, about the third day, seldom later than eight or ten days, after confinement; the chill is attended with feelings of debility, succeeded by a hot fit, with a peculiar kind of headach, a sense of tightness or tension across the forehead, as though it were bound by a cord—at the same time there is a considerable tension, with a soreness, across the lower part of the belly. These characteristic symptoms may occur in different degrees of severity, but they are almost always present. To these symptoms may be added, an altered expression of features, a peculiar vacancy in the expression of the eyes. There is commonly a remission of symptoms each morning, and an aggravation again with the return of the evening.

The lochia (or after discharge) becomes gradually suppressed, and the secretion of milk also disappears.

With the progress of disease the head becomes more and more affected, until delirium supervenes; the patient now sleeps but little, and that little is disturbed; the pulse is rapid, quick and weak, usually one hundred and twenty or more to the minute; frequent sighing; tongue glossy, red and dry; thirst; skin hot and dry, and in the last stages a low muttering delirium, with convulsions.

SUPPRESSION.

Very accurate observation alone can teach us to discriminate, in the first stages, a suppression of lochia, from the commencement of a puerperal fever—nor is it a matter of vital importance should we fail to do so; time alone, in some instances, can settle the question for us. In well-marked cases of suppression we may be more energetic in the use of means to restore the accustomed discharges, and to abate the sufferings of the patient, such as warm applications, mustard, blisters, and opiates, or laudanum and paregoric.

TREATMENT.

From the views already given of the diseased condition of puerperal subjects, it will not be difficult for the reader to comprehend the true indications of cure.

Respect for the opinions of those who advocate the use

of the depletive measures of blood-letting, puking and purging, in the treatment of puerperal fevers, compel us to pass a comment on the chain of reasoning which must lead to such practices; also to state some of the reasons which have brought us to a different conclusion. The existence of pain of head, restlessness, and even frequently delirium, with tumefaction and tenderness of the abdomen, has induced our opponents to infer the existence of what they have been pleased to call inflammation; and when they are fully possessed of that idea, they cannot conceive of any treatment more appropriate than that of abstracting blood, and the use of other active depletive remedies. We have already said, that the philosophy of inflammation has not yet been satisfactorily explained, or that the term is not unfrequently erroneously applied.

When we look to the actual condition of puerperal subjects, and to the natural law in progress, or that should be in progress, to replace the individual back to her former state, or forward to a new and sometimes untried state,—that is, the milk-secreting state,—we find the whole animal economy in a state of great relaxation, and of great exhaustion, from the sudden abstraction of the stimulus of distension, also the escape of more or less of the vital fluids; at the same time the nervous system greatly enfeebled and morbidly sensitive, while the humors are in a state of transition.

Two important phenomena are now taking place, or are about to take place, at one and the same time, viz.: The depurative process, by which the whole genital organs, with their immediate appendages, are reinstating themselves, while the mammæ, or breasts, are engaged in elaborating nourishment for the new being. Under this state of things, we can conceive of congestions, of engorgements of some organs, suppressions of the secretory action of others, and even of a state of what has been termed a sub-acute inflammation; but we cannot conceive of that kind of inflammatory diathesis which calls for the use of the lancet, except it be in young persons, and those, too, of a good constitution and full habits. In such individuals a moderate bleeding might be beneficial in the early stages of the disease. Nauseating remedies, and even emetics, may sometimes be indicated, and sometimes gentle cathartics may be advantageously used. But the chief indication, in our view of the subject, is, to look to the metastasis, or metamorphosis, that is wanted to take place in the natural organic economy, and to afford such aids as are clearly indicated, and no more.

It now remains to show in what way the indications may be met, and the remedial aids applied.

To keep up, or to restore the lochia, and at the same time to allay pain, we use warm fomentations to the abdomen; artificial heat, applied in any way, to the pelvic region, (hips, or lower part of the belly;) mustard plassers; and, in obstinate cases, blisters to the inner and upper parts of the thighs, or to the sides of the abdomen: laudanum, in doses of twenty or thirty drops, to allay pain, procure rest, relieve delirium, and even to relax the patient to the secreting point, which is now suspended by the force of disease.

While these things are in progress, we bring in the aid of the warm bath to the extremities—the warm, diaphoretic teas, to promote the action of the skin, and thereby remove the febrile heat and attendant restlessness.

In order to maintain the tone of the brain and nervous system,—through the instrumentality of which, alone, the equilibrium can be produced and subsisted,—we would give a grain of quinine every hour or two, until the patient is relieved.

Whenever the prostration of the patient is great, the moderate use of some palatable diffusible stimulus, such as wine-whey, sangaree, porteree, toddy, panada, or the like, should be allowed, as an auxiliary to the sustaining influence of the quinine.

BLEEDING.

The earlier practitioners entertained an idea that bleeding should be freely practised; but more modern experience is opposed to it. We have already pointed out the difficulty of reconciling this remedy to the nature and circumstances of the disease. Although we cannot conceive of the existence of a strictly inflammatory diathesis, yet we do conceive that cases may occur, in young and full-habited individuals, in whom the state of congestion, or of inflammation, may be such as to render a moderate bleeding beneficial.

EMETICS.

We are assured, by some respectable practitioners, that this class of remedies, when used at an early stage of the disease, have a decided efficacy; indeed, at one time the French physicians considered them as specifics. Our own personal views, and personal experience, lead us to the belief that they are of more doubtful value than cathartic remedies; or, if they have any useful place in the treatment of puerperal cases, it is in union with other diaphoretic remedies, and only when confined to nauseating potions.

CATHARTICS.

We have in some few cases thought that we witnessed decided salutary effects from the early use of one or more active cathartics; but a more extended experience, and more matured thoughts, have led us to the conclusion that they should not be relied on, and that they should only be used to evacuate improperly retained fœcal matters, or to maintain a natural and salutary state of the bowels.

BLISTERS.

For this class of remedies we have long entertained a partiality, and have used them during the many stages, in the manner before pointed out.

Ever looking to the chain of causation, and to the natural consequence that might be expected to result therefrom, we have never been in favor of much, and especially of active medication of any kind. We have considered it as being one of those conditions of the animal economy in which most good is to be expected from time, rest, management, and the cautious use of mild and slightly modifying agents, to meet particular indications. The type of fever we consider as decidedly typhoid; and in the regular course of the fever would place our chief reliance on the prudent use of small doses of quinine and gentle diaphoretics, so as to excite and to keep up a regular, uniform, but gentle diaphoresis, or sweating. As a sweating and anodyne potion, we have found few agents more efficacious than small doses of camphor and laudanum; say from three to five grains of the former to seven or eight drops of the latter, to be taken every five or six hours. We should by all means endeavor to keep the patient's mind in as confident and cheerful condition as possible.

We have already directed the attention of the reader to a condition of parturient women very closely allied to that of the puerperal state; we mean the simple suppression of the lochia, or the accustomed evacuations from the womb after labour. To relieve the patient of this painful condition, the feet and legs should be well bathed in warm water. To the whole region of the abdomen or belly, or to the hips and back, should warm applications be made with woollen cloths made hot with heated water or otherwise, or by heated bricks or bags of heated sand or salt; while at the same time some twenty-five or thirty-five drops of laudanum, or its equivalent of paregoric, is administered internally, and repeated every two or three hours until the pains abate. When these remedies are used to the extent they should be, it rarely happens that the natural evacuations are not restored in a few hours.

But should this simple course fail to procure the desired change in due time, then you should apply mustard plasters to the insides of the thighs, or even draw blisters with Spanish flies if necessary.

There is still another condition of the parturient female that we should not pass over in silence; we mean after pains: these should be promptly checked by the administration of laudanum, paregoric, or essence of peppermint, and repeated as circumstances required.

DIET.

Patients should be restricted to a light, easily digested, yet sufficiently nutritious diet.

The theoretical doctrines and the practice in the treatment of fevers as pointed out in the foregoing chapters, the author conceives to be so simple, so plain, and at the same time so efficient, that he entertains no doubt but that any common observer, with strict attention, cannot fail to treat all fevers with more success upon his plan than the scientific physician could under the present prejudices in favor of the common or orthodox system of the schools.

This treatise may be justly styled the quinine, or the tonic and diaphoretic practice, admitting of very moderate depletion in the first stage of most fevers, and of the prudent use of stimulants in the last stages of all. The two extremes of depletion and of stimulation, we think must at no distant period meet at this point; and thus reconcile to a great extent the conflicting opinions, the conflicting practices, that have up to this day divided the medical dogmatists of whatever sect, or to whatever schools they may be attached.

CHAPTER XVI.

CONTAINING, IN ALPHABETICAL ORDER, THE CLASSES, OF MEDICINES, WITH AN ACCOUNT OF THE INDIVIDUAL ARTICLES RECOMMENDED IN THIS WORK, THEIR DOSES, USES, AND THE MODES OF ADMINISTERING THEM.

CLASS FIRST.

OF ASTRINGENTS, FROM ASTRINGO, TO BIND.

By this class we understand those articles which, when applied to the body, render the solids denser and firmer, by contracting their fibres independently of their living or muscular powers, and thereby giving strength by counteracting relaxation: such remedies are to be found in both the vegetable and the mineral kingdoms of nature. Their general use is to restrain excessive discharges of any kind from the bowels, womb, or elsewhere. We shall here confine our remarks to those astringents obtained exclusively from the vegetable kingdom.

RUBUS.

(*The root of Blackberry and Dewberry.*)

There are few if any articles of the materia medica affording a more palatable and at the same time useful astringency than the root of the common blackberry or dewberry, (running blackberry). These plants yield their virtues readily to water, and may be used either in a state of warm or cold infusion; its strength should be always proportioned to the age of the patient and the circumstances of the case. The ordinary preparations and mode of preparing for use, is to put from a half to a dozen pieces of root two or three inches long, divested of its outer coat, into a half-pint of water, and taking it as a diet drink, or a few ounces or a common wine-glass full at stated intervals.

After the same manner, and in like cases, the root of the alum-plant, Heuchera Americana, may be used; or the inner bark of any of the family of oaks, querqus, white, black, red, or others, all contain more or less of the gallic acid and of the astringent property.

CEANOTHUS VIRGINIANA.

(*Red-root, New Jersey tea.*)

The root of this shrubby plant, which is to be found in most of the states of this Union, possesses astringent properties worthy of public attention. It may be used for the same purposes that other vegetable astringents are.

LAURUS CINNAMOMUM.

(*Cinnamum-tree.*)

The bark of this tree is possessed of grateful aromatic and slightly astringent properties, and though an article of no great activity as an astringent, it may be found useful in many conditions.

It is used in the form of infusion, or in that of a simple or compound tincture.

Dose of the tincture, one or two drachms.

KINO.
(*A Gum-resin.*)

This is a resinous substance, supposed to be the product of a tree indigenous to the River Gambia, in Africa. It comes to us in resinous masses of a friable nature. It is of a dark red colour. It is one of the most efficacious of the vegetable astringents in use, it may be administered in substance or in the form of tincture, in combination or alone.

Dose in substance from five to twenty grains.—Of the saturated tincture from half a drachm to one drachm or more.

Kino may be advantageously combined with opium, in the proportion of ten grains of the former to one of the latter, or a saturated tincture with paregoric, in equal proportions, or in any proportion to suit the indications of particular cases.

MIMOSA CATECHU.
Extractum Ligni, Catechu, Succus Spissatus. (*The Extract of the Wood.*)

This vegetable extract is brought to us from India; it was formerly called Terra Japanica, or Japan earth. It is possessed of great astringency; it unites a mucilaginous and slightly sweetish taste with that of its astringency.

It is used in the same manner and in about the same doses as the kino.

PAPAVER SOMNIFERUM.
White Poppy.

The capsules, and their inspissated juice, commonly called opium.

Opium, or its most commonly used preparations, laudanum and paregoric, though not properly belonging to the class of astringents, are very useful, and sometimes indispensable remedies in all those fluxes attended with much pain, and may with propriety be united with any of the astringents already spoken of, when the necessity of such a combination is indicated.

The dose of opium, as an astringent, may be from a fourth to a full grain, or more, and should not be repeated oftener than once in four or five hours.

Laudanum is a saturated tincture of opium in whiskey, brandy or rum.

Its dose varies to suit the intentions with which it is used: as an astringent from ten to twenty drops or more; when used to subdue pain, to relieve spasm, and in some cases to procure sleep, we use it in much larger potions.

PAREGORIC ELIXIR.
(Tinctura Opii Camphorata.)

Commonly called camphorated tincture of opium. This is a compound tincture of opium, camphor, flowers of benzoin, and the essential oil of aniseed. It is to be found in the shops under the name of paregoric, or elixir paregoric.

It combines the virtues of the before named articles, and is more manageable in its administration to children, from being more palatable, and, from its dose, containing but one grain of opium to the half ounce, by measure.

The medium dose of paregoric for an adult will be from one to three or four drachms.

We would be guilty of neglect, while recommending the use of opium in its different forms to the public, if we did not at the same time call their attention to the propriety of looking well to the quality of their drugs; also the great importance of using them in their proper doses, for the reason that errors in over-dosing in any of the preparations of opium, are far more dangerous than similar blunders in the doses of any other medicines.

CLASS SECOND.
BLISTERS, OR EXTERNAL IRRITANTS.

This class comprises all those articles which, when applied to the surface of the body, raise or detach the cuticle in the form of vesication, producing serous discharges. They operate as irritants, stimulants, and as drains.

The most common and perhaps the best article now in use for this purpose, is the cantharides or Spanish flies. There are two modes of using them: the one is to confine the pulverized flies in a fine muslin bag, moisten them well with warm vinegar, and confine them to the skin, wherever the blister is intended to be drawn.

The other mode consists in mixing the pulverized flies with any viscid ointment or cerate, and then spreading it into plasters for use.

The sizes of blister plasters should be proportioned to the ages and sizes of individuals, to the intentions with which they are used, as also to the parts of the body to which they may be applied; the medium size for an adult being about three or four inches square.

There are many other articles that may be used for the same purpose, and in the same way. The best known substitute for Spanish flies is the Lytta Vittata, or potatoe fly, which may be treated and used as above directed.

The black and the white mustard seed, when ground and applied to the skin, promptly inflames and even excites vesication. Its greater promptitude of action and comparative little liability to detach the cuticle, in many instances give it a preference over the blistering flies.

There are many other articles which act as stimulants and irritants when applied to the skin, such as the inner bark of the white walnut, (Juglans Cenerea,) the blister weed, and some others.

Blisters should be invariably clipped, and the effused serum suffered to escape so soon as they have drawn or filled, otherwise the patient is in danger of that distressing affection of the neck of the bladder, called stranguary.— They should be dressed with coddled plantain, or cabbage leaves, or some suitable cerate.

CLASS THIRD.
OF INTERNAL IRRITANTS, OR EMETICS, CATHARTICS AND INJECTIONS, OR CLYSTERS.

Words being used as the signs or representatives of things, or of ideas, are ever more or less arbitrary in themselves, while they are made to vary in their significations to suit the purposes of different minds, or minds entertaining different views on the same subject or the same thing. We find ourselves under the necessity of doing one of two things, either to coin new terms, or to affix a varied and in some respects a new signification to old words. Hence, that which most writers have been pleased to call local stimulants, we have thought fit to denominate internal irritants.

By the use of this term we mean to convey the idea of such articles as, taken inwardly, irritate or derange the natural action of the living fibre, either by increase, diminution, or departure from its natural play.

We call emetics, cathartics and clysters, irritants, for the reason that we conceive their action to result from an effort of nature to remove them or to cast them off; while to the term stimulants proper, we have attached the idea of articles congenial to the animal economy, and acting in unison with its laws.

SECTION FIRST.
OF EMETICS.

Emetics are those medicines that excite vomiting, independently of any effect arising from their mere bulk.

CŒPHALIS IPECACUANHA.

Ipecacuan, Ipecac. (*The Pulverized Root.*)

There is no one article of this class of remedies better entitled to claims for its safety and usefulness than that of ipecac. The experience of most practitioners has led them to give it a preference over any other article of its class, especially when introduced in the treatment of febrile diseases.

It is administered in substance, in doses of from ten to twenty, or more grains. It should be mixed in warm water, and given in divided portions; say one-fourth every fifteen or twenty minutes, until its effects are produced. A more pleasant way of using it is that of the vinous tincture, usually kept in the shops under the name of ipecac. wine. The dose of this preparation depends, in some measure, on the solvent property of the wine; it usually requires a half-ounce, or more, for an adult—one or more tea-spoonfulls to puke a child.

LOBELIA INFLATA.

Emetic Weed. Indian Tobacco. The Leaves.

This is an annual plant, indigenous to many parts of the United States. Of late years, its virtues have been much, perhaps too much eulogised, by the Thompsonians and others. Dose, of the powdered leaves, from ten to twenty grains; of the saturated tincture, one or more drachms.

TARTAR EMETIC.

The properties of this drug have long been known to the people. It ranks among the most active of the class to which it belongs. Its dose is from one to four or five grains. It should always be used in warm water, and in broken doses, at intervals of fifteen or twenty minutes.

Emetic medicines should always be administered in warm water, and in divided portions; and after each fit of puking, a portion of warm water, some warm tea, or gruel, should be given, to promote its action on the stomach, skin or bowels, as may be desired.

No cold drinks, of any kind, should be indulged in, until its operation is completely over.

SECTION SECOND.
CATHARTICS.

We come, next, to the consideration of those medicines which, taken internally, increase the natural expulsive action of the bowels.

RICINUS COMMUNIS.
Palma Christi, Ricinus. Castor Oil.

The expressed oil of the seed of the palma christi plant has, of late years, become an article of very general use, and is always to be found in the shops of those who trade in medicines. The certainty and mildness of its operations make it particularly well adapted to the cases of children. Its dose, for an adult, is from half-an-ounce to an ounce or more.

CASSIA SENNA—SENNA.
The Leaves.

Of this article there are several kinds commonly to be found in the shops. The Alexandrian and the Italian is most generally met with. It is a useful cathartic, operating mildly, yet efficiently. The most convenient mode of administering it is that of infusion.

From two to six drachms of the leaves to the half-pint, or more, of boiling water; to be taken in divided portions, so as not to oppress the stomach. It is also used in the form of tincture, and of compound tincture.

RHEUM PALMATUM.
Rhubarb. The Root.

This is a mild purgative; operates without violence or irritation, and may be given with safety to pregnant women and to children. Its dose, for an adult, is about twenty or thirty grains. It may be used in infusion, in tincture, or in combination with other cathartics.

CONVOLVULUS JALAPA.
Jalap. The Root.

This article has been long in use; it is an effectual, and generally a safe purgative. Dose, from ten to twenty grains. It may be taken alone, or in union with other cathartic drugs. It is used, also, in the form of simple and compound tincture,

ALOE PERFOLIATA GUMMI RESINA.

Barbadoes, or Hepatic and Socoterine Aloes.

Aloes is a bitter and stimulating, or heating purgative; its impressions are chiefly made on the lower intestines. In doses of from five to fifteen grains it empties the large intestines, without making the stools thin. Emmenagogue virtues are ascribed to it. It is most commonly used in combination with other cathartics, in the form of pills; indeed, it constitutes an important item in most of the purgative nostrums. It is used in many compound purgative tinctures.

The neutral salts afford us many gentle and useful purgatives.

SULPHAS MAGNESIA.

Sulphate of Magnesia. Epsom Salts.

This is a mild and gentle purgative, yet operating with sufficient activity. It should be administered in warm water. Dose, six or eight drachms.

SUPER-TARTRIS POTASSÆ.

Super Tartrate of Potass, Crystals of Tartar, and Cream of Tartar.

This is a gentle and cooling purgative. Dose, from half-an-ounce to an ounce or more. When given in smaller doses, it often acts as a diuretic.

SUB-MURIAS HYDRARGYRI.

Sub-muriate of Quicksilver. Formerly Calomel. (Calomel.)

Calomel has long been in common use, and is justly considered one of the best mercurial preparations we possess. By proper management, it may be made to answer many valuable purposes. It may be made to increase almost any of the secretions, or excretions. Given in doses of one grain, night and morning, or even in larger doses, united with a little opium, or some astringent, to prevent it from running off by the bowels, it excites ptyalism [salivation.] In doses of from five to twenty grains, it is an effectual and excellent purgative. In small and repeated doses of two or three grains, taken at intervals of two or three days, it is thought to have a powerful and salutary effect in relieving obstructions, and chronic inflammations of the abdominal viscera generally, and especially of the liver.

There is another mercurial preparation now much used, and by many practitioners preferred to calomel, (we mean the blue mass.) As an alterative, it is given in one or two grain doses; as a purgative, from four to six or eight grains.

SECTION THIRD.
OF INJECTIONS OR CLYSTERS.

This is still another mode of bringing remedies to act on the internal surfaces, called surfaces of relation. Clysters are commonly used to evacuate the larger and lower intestines. But clysters or injections may be either irritating, stimulating, evacuating, soothing, astringent, or even nutritious, to answer the various purposes for which they may be designed. In cases of fever, however, they are very rarely used, except to obviate costiveness, or to restrain undue evacuations from the bowels.

Clysters, when used to evacuate the bowels of persons who are feeble and confined by fever, should be very mild only rendered active enough to answer the purposes intended. The following are cheap and convenient modes of preparing them.

To a pint of thin broth or gruel, add two table spoonfuls of sugar or molasses, or to the same amount of gruel simply add one table spoonful of table salt, or of Epsom salts, or castor oil, or you may use common hog's lard in lieu of the salts or oil; any one of these formulas makes a mild, cheap, and effectual injection. The composition thus made ready for injecting should be brought to the temperature of the body before it is introduced. Should it fail to operate, or not operate effectually, then should the activity of the injection be increased, or the process repeated every three or four hours, until the object for which it was intended is accomplished.

Injections are sometimes needed to allay pain, or to restrain evacuations from the bowels. In such cases from twenty to sixty drops of laudanum, to suit the indications of the case, in a few ounces of sweet milk, or a mucilage of starch or gum arabic constitutes a suitable injection, or when the indications are merely to restrain a looseness of the bowels, then any of the astringent effusions may be used

CLASS FOURTH.

OF GENERAL STIMULANTS, OR STIMULANTS PROPER, INCLUDING NARCOTICS AND ANTI-SPASMODICS.

By this class of remedies we understand such articles as, when taken inwardly, promptly pervade the whole system, and which act either by exalting the natural action of the brain and nervous system, or by retarding the consumption of the natural elements of life, according to the particular article used, and to the condition and circumstances of the individual at the time being.

This class in these phenomena displaying a marked distinction from what are called by many writers local stimulants, or what we have thought fit to style irritants, the modus operandi of stimulants must ever vary with the condition of the living economy in which they are received; while endless varieties of shades and grades of phenomena result from the administration of the different elements or articles that compose this extended class, no two articles possessing identically the same virtues.

The appreciable or demonstrable difference in the properties of the numerous articles used as manifested by their action on the animal economy, has given rise to the common classification or division of general stimulants into the heads called narcotics, anti-spasmodics, anodyne, and so forth. We shall consider them all under one and the same head, namely, that of general stimulants.

The characteristic distinctions which we conceive to exist between these two grand divisions of the materia medica, viz., *stimulants* and *irritants*, consists in the fact, that the one class of agents tends to exalt, to tranquilize, and to sustain the vital energies, while the other invariably tends to deplete, to evacuate, and to waste.

We have already contended for the efficacy and salubrity of that portion of diffusible stimulants usually called luxuries, viz.: wine, cider, the malt liquors, rum, whiskey, brandy, and their subdivisions. Now, any one of these articles, under the guidance of wisdom, may be made to answer a valuable purpose in certain diseased conditions of the animal economy. They may be made to sustain life, to promote animal heat, to allay pain, and to counteract spasm.

The truth is, that a great portion of our bodily pains arise from a want of action, a defect in the natural excitement of the structure which is the seat of pain.

There is ever the same discriminating judgment required in the administration of stimulants, that there is in the use of depletive measures.

In the treatment of fevers, it ever has been an important point to know where the use of depletives should terminate, and the introduction of stimulants should begin. In the use of stimulants, then, we should ever be guarded: commence with small potions, and vigilantly watch their effects. Our practice has been with the distilled liquors, to commence with table spoonful doses put in the most palatable form, and repeated every three or four hours. Wines and malt liquors should be used in larger quantities.

LAURUS CAMPHORA.
(Camphor-tree, Camphor.)

This is a peculiar vegetable product, of a white, crystalline appearance, nearly transparent, concrete, and friable, taste bitter and acrid, smell penetrating and peculiar.

The camphor of commerce is obtained from the camphor-tree of Japan by distillation; the thyme, rosemary, sage, peppermint, and some other plants afford the same principle in small quantities.

Camphor is an active substance when taken into the stomach. It increases the heat of the body, produces a tendency to diaphoresis, but without quickening the pulse.

It has been found useful in all languid and depressed conditions of the body.

Stimulant, antiseptic, anodyne, and diaphoretic virtues have been ascribed to it.

It should be administered either in a spirituous or vinous solution, or in a state of minute mechanical division. A convenient form of administering it is to triturate with a little spirit of any kind, or with sugar and milk.

Dose from three to five grains or more. Three grains of camphor with seven or eight drops of laudanum, constitute a useful diaphoretic in low grades of fever. The dose should be repeated once in five or six hours.

SPIRITUS AMMONIA AROMATICUS.
(*Aromatic Spirit of Ammonia, or Compound Spirit of Ammonia.*)

In this preparation we have the spirit of ammonia or hartshorn united with aromatics, which renders its flavor more agreeable and acceptable to the stomach than the uncombined spirit would be. It may be used as a simple stimulant, and is sometimes found beneficial to check vomitings. Dose one drachm, or more.

TINCTURA LAVENDULÆ COMPOSITA.
(*Compound Spirit of Lavender.*)

The compound spirit of lavender is a grateful cordial, well calculated to allay irritation of the stomach, and to restrain operations from either stomach or bowels: its dose is from a half to one or more drachms.

OPIUM.

Of this article we have already spoken at some length under the head of astringents; it is here proper that we should speak of it as a stimulant and as an anodyne; when used with a view merely to stimulate, it should be used in small doses and at short intervals. When used with a view to allay pain, or to procure sleep, it should be used in larger doses, and at longer intervals.

CLASS FIFTH.

OF DIAPHORETICS OR SUDORIFICS.

Under this head we shall consider some of those means and those remedies which taken inwardly promote the natural discharges from the surface of the body.

The skin being one of the natural and constant waste ways of the body, any interruption to the performance of its natural functions, is quickly followed by signs of distress, or deranged action in the animal economy; hence the great importance in the treatment of febrile diseases, of understanding the functions of the skin, and regulating its action.

The circumstances most favorable for the action of diaphoretics, is a warm atmosphere, or warm clothing, the free use of diluents, quietude, and in many conditions sleep. In cases where a free and protracted diaphoresis is desired, the plentiful use of diluents must be allowed, since they are necessary to maintain the requisite fluidity of the blood, through which alone a diaphoresis can be sustained.

There are many simple vegetable teas which, when taken moderately strong, and continued for some hours under favorable circumstances, produce decided diaphoretic effects. We will mention some of them in the order in which they stand in our estimation.

ARISTOLOCHIA SERPENTARIA.

(Serpentaria Virginiana, Virginia Snake-root.)

This article may be considered a slightly stimulating tonic, diaphoretic. It has been found useful in some stages of most fevers, and to bring out the eruption in eruptive diseases, either when the eruption is tardy in making its appearance, or has receded; it also sometimes constitutes a good auxiliary in the cure of intermittent fevers. Its dose in substance is from ten to twenty or thirty grains, but it is in the form of infusion that it is mostly used. The proportions are a pint of boiling water to the half ounce of the dried root. Of this infusion one or two fluid ounces should be taken every two or three hours. In a similar way, with slight changes in the proportions or doses, may any of the following articles be used viz.:

The European or American pennyroyal, mentha pulegium, saffron, crocus sativus, sassafras, laurus sassafras, common hyssop, hyssopi officinalis, sage, salvia officinalis, balm, melessa officinalis.

PULVIS IPECACUANHA ET OPII.

(Compound Powder of Ipecac. and Opium, Dover's Powder.)

This powder is composed of opium and ipecac. each one part, and sulphate or nitrate of potash eight parts. This preparation constitutes a very useful and popular remedy. Its dose is from five to ten or fifteen grains diffused in water or mixed in syrup, and repeated at intervals of four, six, or eight hours. Opium united with camphor in the proportion of a fourth of a grain of the former to three quarters of the latter, will be found admissible in many cases where the Dover's Powder cannot be used on account of its nauseating effect.

SPIRITUS ÆTHERIS NITRICI.

(Sweet Spirit of Nitre.)

The sweet spirit of nitre is extensively employed in febrile affections for the purpose of exciting the secretions, especially those of the kidneys and skin. Its dose varies from a half to one or more drachms, given every two or three hours.

OF THE ALKALINE DIAPHORETICS.

The supercarbonates or bicarbonates of potash and of

soda are justly entitled to a place among the sweating remedies used in the treatment of fevers. These alkalies may be used in some of the mild herb teas or in simple cool water. Dose of either preparation from ten to fifty or sixty grains.

The citric or acetous acid, that is, lemon acid, or vinegar united with the carbonates of potash, soda or ammonia to the point of saturation, makes good diaphoretic mixtures, commonly called saline mixtures.

CLASS SEVENTH.

OF TONICS.

We come now to the consideration of that class of remedies which in our humble estimation claims the first rank in the treatment of fevers. Tonics, in a general sense, include every thing which invigorates the powers of life; while in a more limited, in a medicinal sense, it implies such substances as are exhibited to correct debility. Of their modus operandi the limits of this treatise will not permit us fully to speak. Suffice it to say, that the effects of all real tonics, when rightly used, are to impart tone and energy to the brain, the nervous, and muscular systems; to maintain the proper degree of animal heat without running it to excess, to improve the powers of digestion, and to promote the functional duties of all the organic structure.

We shall first take into consideration some of the vegetable tonics, and close this article by some remarks on mineral tonics. At the head of this class of remedies we have thought fit to place cinchona.

CINCHONA.

(Cinchona Flava, Yellow Bark. Cinchola Palida, Pale Bark. Cinchona Rubra, Red Bark.)

Although the Peruvian Bark was introduced into Europe as early as sixteen hundred and forty, and has continued to be prescribed by physicians ever since, yet still it is but recently that its virtues seem to have been fully appreciated, or its modus operandi on the animal economy to have been comprehended.

One important era in the history of its usefulness, is marked by the researches of Pelletier and Caventau, who first succeeded by a chemical process in extracting its salt or its alkaline element, in which its virtues principally reside, called cinchonine, or quinine. Another era in its history has been more recently marked by the labors of Professor Liebig, who, in his investigations of organic chemistry, endeavors to show the relationship that exists between this particular salt and the human brain and nervous tissues, and thereby suggesting an explanation of its efficacy and of its mode of operating on the animal economy.

Almost all enlightened practitioners, of this or other countries, concur in ascribing to quinine, or the active matter of Peruvian bark, the virtues of a tonic, antiseptic, and even febrifuge. About its tonic and antiseptic properties, there seems to be but little discrepancy; it is as to the extent of its febrifuge qualities that a collision of thought may arise. We have taken the position, based on personal experience, that quinine is not only admissible, but it is in truth the most efficient febrifuge known to us in almost all stages of all fevers proper, and we leave to time, and the experience of others, to settle the truth of the position.

Under the different heads of fevers, and other diseases treated of in this work, we have already indicated the circumstances in which it should be administered; it here only remains for us to point out the forms and doses in which it should be used. Quinine may be administered either in substance, with a little sugar or syrup, of any kind, or in solution.

When used in substance, the following is the author's formula:

R. Sulphate of quinine,...................40 grains.
   Gum myrrh,..........................10 "
   Liquorice,............................30 "

Triturate well; moisten with a little water, and add just enough of the oil of sassafras to impart an agreeable odor: Divide into forty pills; each pill then contains, of quinine, one grain; of myrrh, one-fourth of a grain; of liquorice, three-fourths of a grain. Dose, one pill: to be repeated every one or two hours, or longer, to suit the case.

FORMULA FOR A SOLUTION OF QUININE.

Take of sulphate of quinine,............16 grains.
Of whiskey, or other spirit, or water,.....2 ounces.

Add as many drops of elixir of vitriol, or sulphuric acid, as will render the quinine soluble. The elixir of vitriol, or sulphuric acid, is not necessary, if the vial is always well shaken just before pouring out a dose. This solution contains one grain of quinine to the drachm: its dose, then, is a tea-spoonful, or one drachm. This is the most convenient form for administering to children. The dose is readily reduced to suit the ages of children, and can be made palatable by the addition of sugar and water.

We have here, as elsewhere, indicated the medium doses in which quinine should be used. Our own experience, and the experience of others, go to show, that no danger or bad consequences are to be apprehended from much larger doses than we have used.*

There are many other vegetables endowed with valuable tonic properties, both foreign and indigenous, and which, in the hands of different practitioners, have obtained various reputations for usefulness. We will mention a few of them,—principally natives,—for the reason, that it should

---

* As the druggists and physicians, in all probability, will purchase and send out pills and drops, purporting to be compounded of quinine of the proper strength, and which may not contain one-fourth the quantity of this article they should contain, and thereby defeat the object we intend, we would advise each family to procure the quinine at the stores, or apothecaries', as they do their sugar, coffee, or tea; and to prepare it themselves, as recommended in this treatise.

be an object with every one to know the best substitute that our own country can afford for the cinchona:

>Cornus Florida, dog-wood.
>Cornus sericea, swamp dog-wood.
>The inner bark—bark of the root.

The bark of these native trees was first brought into notice by Dr. Walker, of Virginia. It is still in common use with the country people as a tonic bitter, and is sometimes used to cure intermittents. It has been thought by many a good substitute for the cinchona officinalis.

Prunus Virginiana, or Wild Cherry.

The inner bark of the common wild cherry, either pulverized, or used in decoction or infusion, has long been a popular remedy with many for the cure of intermittents and other diseases.

It has been found best to unite the bark of the dog-wood with that of the cherry tree.

COLOMBA, COLOMBO.

Calculus Palmatus. The Root.

Also, the American Columbo; the Frasera Walteri. The roots of these plants, both the foreign and the native columba, have been found useful, mild tonics, and have been used in intermittents, and recommended in the declining stages of remittent fevers. Used either in substance or in infusion. The dose of the dried root is from ten to thirty grains, three or four times, or oftener, per day.

There are some other indigenous plants, which we think more justly entitled to our notice than any of those already mentioned; we mean that family called by the botanists eupatorium.

EUPATORIUM PERFOLIATUM.

Thoroughwort, Indian Sage. Bone-set, the Leaves.

The virtues of this plant are said to have been known

to the Indians. By them it was used in the cure of intermittents, and other diseases. We have had some experience in its use, and consider it one of the best native vegetable tonics known; and think that, in all probability, it may be found to supply the place of the cinchona more effectually than any other of the numerous American tonics. It may be used in substance, in extract, or in infusion. Dose, of the powdered leaves, twenty or thirty grains.

The eupatorium should be used in moderate portions, when used as a tonic; as it is apt, when administered in large doses, to excite puking or purging.

There is another native plant called black-root, Boman, Brenton or Albulver's physic, which is endowed with virtues equal, and in many respects similar, to those of the eupatorium perfoliatum. Its virtues reside, principally, in the root. Dose: The black-root should be used in the same way, and in about the same doses, as the eupatorium perfoliatum.*

MINERAL TONICS, OR DURABLE TONICS.

The mineral as well as the vegetable kingdom, affords us some valuable tonics. We shall not go into an estimate of the comparative value of the different minerals used as tonic remedies; but shall notice only some of those that we consider to be the most durable, and most congenial to the animal economy.

FERRUM, OR IRON.

Many of the preparations of iron have been long in use as tonics, and they have been supposed more congenial to

---

* The author is of opinion, from his own experience, that either of these two plants is greatly preferable to any of the indigenous tonics mentioned; and that either of them, when properly used, will be found a pretty good substitute for the quinine, as well in the prevention as in the cure of fevers.

animal life than other metals, for the reason that it alone of all the metals constitutes an element in our structure.

FERRI CARBONAS PRECIPITATUS.

Precipitated Carbonate of Iron.

The precipitated carbonate of iron differs but little from that carbonate commonly called the rust of iron, the chief difference being in the manner of preparing.

The carbonate of iron is an excellent and safe chalybeate; it may be considered as the most permanent of all the tonics, and is well adapted to the treatment of many chronic diseases.

Dose, from five to fifty or sixty grains.

The preparations of iron answer better in small doses, frequently repeated, than in large doses. The carbonate of iron is conveniently administered in honey, molasses, or syrup of any kind.

FERRI ACETAS.

Acetate of Iron.

This is a saturated solution of iron in vinegar. The scales of iron, the filings, or the carbonate, may be used for this preparation. It is equally beneficial and active as other preparations of iron.

The dose will depend on the strength of the acid employed. From half a drachm to a drachm is the common dose, taken in a little water or other suitable vehicle.

CLASS VII.

VERMIFUGES, OR ANTHELMINTICS.

Vermifuges are such medicines as procure the evacuation of worms from the stomach and intestines. We shall only speak of those articles that we have found most uniformly successful.

CHENOPODIUM ANTHELMINTICUM.

Worm-Seed. Jerusalem Oak.

This article, as a vermifuge, has long been in general use; the whole plant may be employed. The expressed juice of the green leaves, a decoction of the plant, or the seed taken in lozenges, or otherwise; its virtues reside in its essential oil—hence the oil of worm-seed is the most active preparation.

Dose, for an adult about twenty drops or more of the oil, two or three times a day.

SPIGELIA, PINK ROOT.

Spigelia Marylandica.

The vermifuge properties of this plant are said to have been first learned from the Cherokee Indians. The remedy certainly stands high in this country as an anthelmintic; it has also been recommended in infantile remittents, and other febrile diseases.

It may be given in substance or infusion. The dose in substance is from one to two drachms, to be repeated morning and evening, for several days successively, and then followed by a cathartic. Spigelia constitutes the active matter in most of the worm nostrums, called worm syrups, worm powders, and worm teas.

The success of vermifuges will be greatly facilitated by attention to the condition of the bowels. After using the worm medicine for a day or two, if the bowels are not sufficiently open, then some suitable cathartic should be directed, such as a dose of calomel, a portion of castor oil, or senna, so as to promote the expulsion of the worms.

After taking children through a course of worm medicines, they should invariably be put on the use of some bitter tonics, once or twice a day, until their general health and strength is restored.

WEIGHTS AND MEASURES.

That the general reader may the better comprehend the correct administration of the different remedies recommended in this treatise, we have thought fit to insert the following tables, viz.:

TABLE OF APOTHECARIES' WEIGHT.

POUND,	OUNCES,	DRACHMS,	SCRUPLES,	GRAINS.
1	12	96	288	5,760
0	1	8	24	480
0	0	1	3	60
0	0	0	1	20

For convenience we often direct medicines to be taken by the measurement of certain household implements, but it is necessary that we have definite ideas attached to them.

A teacup is estimated to contain about four fluid ounces, or a gill.
A wine-glass " " " two fluid ounces.
A table-spoon " " " half a fluid ounce.
A tea-spoon " " " a fluid drachm.

Since in the body of this treatise we have seldom spoken of the doses of the different remedies recommended, except in reference to adults, we have thought it advisable to present some general rule by which the practitioner or attendant will be the better enabled to proportion the doses of medicines to the ages of his patients. For this purpose we have adopted the following table of Gaubious, which has received the approbation of many experienced practitioners.

TABLE OF GAUBIOUS.

The dose for a person of middle age being one, or one measure or quantity of any kind, one drachm, or 60 grains; for example:—

That of a person from
14 to 21 years of age will be ⅔ or 2 scruples, or 40 grains.
7 to 14 "   "   " ½ or ½ drachm, or 30 grains.
4 to 7 "   "   " ⅓ or 1 scruple, or 20 grains.
Of 4 "   "   " ¼ or 15 grains.
3 "   "   " ⅙ or 10 grains.
2 "   "   " ⅛ or 8 grains.
1 "   "   " 1/12 or 5 grains.

In like manner, when one grain constitutes a dose for an adult, of any article, (quinine for example,) then it should be reduced to parts of a grain, to suit the ages of children, according to the rule laid down in the above table.

The foregoing table of Gaubious is intended as a general rule by which to scale down any or all the articles of the materia medica, to suit the different ages of patients; but we think it would be well to remark, that experience has taught us, that in some articles we may vary from the proportions indicated in the table; for example—castor oil is given in ounce doses to adults, while we give one or two teaspoonsful to children under one year old, and even when but a few weeks old; while in the administration of laudanum, we should not depart from the rule—for example—if we take 24 or 26 drops as a medium dose for an adult, then the one-twelfth, or two drops, will suffice for a child one year old.

The result of the author's experience in the administration of quinine goes to show that it should be administered in larger portions to young persons than the rule laid down by the table would direct; that is to say, in administering the solution of quinine, made after his formula, (containing one grain to the drachm, or teaspoonful,) he has successfully administered it to persons of the following ages, in about the following proportions, viz:

A person from
12 to 16 years of age will take from 60 to 100 drops.
8 to 12 "   "   "   "   " 30 to 40 "
4 to 8 "   "   "   "   " 15 to 30 "
1 to 4 "   "   "   "   " 8 to 15 "
An infant under one year "   "   " 3 to 8 "

A drachm of the solution of quinine contains about 110 drops.

The author of the foregoing pages, in writing out his views on the theory and treatment of fevers, has found himself compelled to retain some of the technicalities of the schools; but whenever he has done so, he has given an explanation of their meaning. In giving an account of the medicines recommended, he has thought it best to retain all of the names in common use either with apothecaries or others, for the reason that different individuals were in the habit of calling the same articles by different names. The technical terms made use of by the different writers from whom we have made quotations, we do not feel at liberty to explain.

APPENDIX.

A Report of a singular Case of Stone in the Bladder, occurring in the Practice of the Author.

On the fifteenth day of June, 1823, I was requested to ride twenty-five miles to visit a negro girl, about fifteen years old, who had swallowed a very large sewing needle, eighteen months or two years previous to that time, and who had complained of some uneasiness in the stomach and bowels from the time of swallowing it; but for much the greater part of the time had suffered excruciating pain in and about her privates.

It was expected that I could ascertain where the needle was, and by some means extract it.

Upon external examination I found no point to warrant an operation, and determined to examine per vaginam. On introducing my finger, I found a hard substance occupying a large portion of the pelvis. I then introduced a sound into the bladder, and contrary to all expectation, met with a stone as large as a goose egg.

She was emaciated in the extreme; but as she and her master were both desirous of having an operation performed at all hazards, I proceeded to operate by introducing a sharp-pointed curved bistoury, as high up into the bladder as I thought necessary and proper—the index finger of my left hand being up the vagina, so as to meet its point, and to act as a guard; the one incision was sufficient.

I then introduced a pair of strong forceps (made that day,) to break up the stone; but from some cause not then known to me, I found it impossible to pass the forceps as high up as I wished and expected; I however broke off about one-third part of it, and extracted it by piecemeal, expecting the balance would advance and occupy the place of that which had been removed. In that, however, I was disappointed; it was stationary. I then made several fruitless attempts to fasten the forceps upon the stone. I had pressure made on the lower part of the belly to assist in advancing it, and to keep the parts more steady, but all to no purpose—for the forceps could not take hold on it.

I then passed my finger up into the bladder, and found that the remaining part of the stone was partially enveloped by and firmly attached to the bladder, the separation of which required all the force I could exert with my finger, but ultimately succeeded by alternately skinning as it were the bladder with my finger, and then breaking down or scaling off the stone with the forceps.

Until I had removed the greater part of the stone, I thought it was a mistake about her having swallowed the needle at all; or that, if she had, it had by some means escaped unnoticed; but on finding the point near the centre of the stone, the eye of which might not have passed to the inner part of the bladder, all doubts were dispelled.

The needle was extracted, the balance of the stone removed, and the bladder carefully examined, so that no fragment of the stone should be left adhering to it, and the parts well syringed, and all extraneous particles removed.

The patient was then put to bed, and an anodyne draught given her. On seeing her the next morning, I found her quite cheerful, she had no pain nor soreness, except when she moved in bed. Her recovery was rapid, and she enjoyed good health as long as the family remained in the neighborhood. But, as is common after such an operation, she laboured under a partial inability to retain her urine.

Different opinions have been entertained relative to the spontaneous or non-spontaneous productions of vegetable and animal substances, or whether, at any time, or under any circumstances, these substances are produced by a mere combination of circumstances, such as a certain condition of the earth, acted on by the sun, and air, &c., independent of any seed or germ.

It has also been a subject of much speculation among physicians how calculous concretions are formed in the gall-bladder, urinary bladder, and elsewhere. It is contended by some that there must be a seed, a germ or nucleus for the formation of stone in those parts, while others adhere to the opinion that from the mere nature, tendency and propension of the secretions, stony concretions are produced.

Whatever may be the cause of the formation of stone in the bladder, or whatever may be the opinion of physicians upon the subject, I am well assured in the present case, that the needle was the nucleus around which this immense mass of stony matter was formed.

I have published this case more from its novelty than from any benefit that it is expected society may derive from it, as it is probable that precisely such a case never did occur before, and never may again.

ASIATIC CHOLERA.

A few Remarks on the Character and Treatment of Asiatic Spasmodic or Epidemic Cholera.

This disease has carried terror and desolation wherever it has gone, perhaps more than any other disease. It was not confined to any climate, nor to any particular season of the year; in our country, however, it was most common in the summer and fall seasons of the year, raging chiefly in large cities, towns, and on navigable streams, and other places where there was the greatest concourse of people. Like some other epidemics, it had its origin in the oldest inhabited and most eastern part of the globe, and seemed to have required sixteen or eighteen years to travel to the far west. In this particular it seems but to have followed in the footsteps of man, who in his migration has ever moved from east to west.

It seems most probable that it was of atmospheric origin, in some way or other predisposing the system to the disease, and that fear was sometimes the exciting cause I have but little doubt. In the strict sense of the word, I do not believe it to have been a contagious disease, but like some other diseases, when the system was impregnated with the poison, or the predisposing cause, breathing the limited atmosphere of the sick, especially where sufficient ventilation and cleanliness were not observed, or suffering very unpleasant and fearful associations of the mind, all acted as exciting causes.

Both sexes were equally subject to it, when they had arrived at or passed the age of puberty; nor can I say that habit or peculiarity of constitution made a marked difference in its effects, but so far as it came under my observation, children were entirely exempted from it.

SYMPTOMS.

The premonitory symptoms, when such were recognised, were a mild looseness of the bowels, and decline of appetite, with scarcely any other indisposition; this state of things was of various duration, depending upon the presence or absence of exciting causes.

In some instances, the looseness continued for several days before the characteristic symptoms of the disease supervened; in other cases its duration was for a few hours only, and occasionally the first intimation of the attack was a sudden and extremely free discharge from the bowels, unaccompanied with pain, the patient feeling as if the whole contents of the bowels were passing off at once, as in reality was sometimes the case.

But suddenly there is a re-accumulation of fluid in the intestines, by the inverted action of the absorbents of the stomach and bowels.

Sometimes the attack came on with sick stomach and vomiting, without any looseness of the bowels. But whether the premonitory symptoms of looseness of the bowels continued a longer or a shorter time, or whether there was none at all, whenever these copious discharges of chyle and serum began to flow, that is, the rice-water or milk-like discharges, made their appearance, then it might be considered a confirmed case of cholera, of more or less intensity, in proportion to the frequency and quantity of the discharges. General and most distressing cramps were apt to follow: soon, though not always, a death-like coldness of the skin supervened.

Profuse cold sweats now came on, the breath and tongue are cold, the skin assumes a dark brown or livid hue, and becomes shrunk, as though it had been for several hours immersed in water, especially about the hands, feet, and face; their features are so changed in a few hours, that their most intimate acquaintances will scarcely know them; their eyes are sunk and haggard, the pulse often sinks in an hour or two so that it is not perceivable at the wrists; there is a great sense of inward heat and thirst. During the whole course of the disease, there is very rarely any discharge of bile or of urine. While the skin of the patient is as cold as marble, he is apt to complain of an unpleasant sensation of heat, when external warmth is applied to him. Delirium is a rare occurrence in cholera.

The foregoing are the common symptoms of cholera, nor should it be a matter of surprise that the symptoms should run their course in such rapid succession upon one another, since the chyle and serum, that is, the fluid elements of the blood, and the nutritious principle of the body, are running off in streams from the stomach and bowels, as well as from the whole surface of the body through the pores of the skin.

As soon as these rice-water or milk-and-water-like discharges begin to flow, and which are sometimes among the earliest discoverable symptoms, other symptoms may or may not accompany them; or if they do, they follow in such rapid succession, that often in an hour or two, the whole of them are seen running to the lowest possible point, the whole system is regularly and rapidly collapsing, until the patient either dies, or the disease is arrested.

If the disease be not arrested, either by nature or by art, it generally runs its course in from 6 to 24, or 48 hours, varying in proportion to the severity of the attack.

The general symptoms of Asiatic cholera are for the most part uniform, that is, there is a sameness in the characteristic features of the disease, consequently the general indications of cure are pretty much the same, unless indeed, as happens in some cases and in some seasons, consecutive fevers supervene; but this never takes place until the cholera symptoms begin to subside.

There are surely not many subjects upon which misguided education, or sectarian principles, or dogmas are more plainly and injuriously manifested, than in the theory and practice in the disease now under consideration.

Asiatic cholera is unquestionably a disease from its commencement, and throughout its whole course entirely divested of what is called an inflammatory diathesis. On the contrary there is evidently a want of tonic action, which cannot be misunderstood by any unprejudiced mind, from the symptoms and circumstances attendant on it. The skin is cold, the arterial action extremely feeble, sometimes not even perceptible at the wrists; and to these signs of prostration and relaxation, may be added, life is running from the patient in sluices, by excessive discharges of chyle and serum, from an inverted action of the absorbents of the stomach and bowels, and by profuse, cold, clammy sweats, from the whole surface of the body. The patient is, at the same time, prostrated by the most painful spasms.

Yet, strange as it may appear, under all these circumstances, and signs of exhaustion, of a wasting disease, there are physicians to be found,—men, too, who claim to be orthodox practitioners,—who advise free bleeding, active puking and purging; while others, of high standing, not concurring in the practice of such marked depletion, recommend the sedative influence of cold drinks and ice-water. It is recorded of some that they opened the jugular veins and temporal arteries of their patients; while others gave a pound of calomel in the course of forty-eight hours.—[See Eberle, vol. ii., page 558, on spasmodic cholera.] Here are 4320 grains of the most insidious poison in the materia medica given to one patient in the course of twenty-four hours!

We have known several of our western brethren who administered calomel in table-spoonful doses; that is, about six hundred and sixty grains to the dose.

AN ACCOUNT OF THE PERSONAL EXPERIENCE OF THE AUTHOR.

In the summer of 1833, the first case of cholera occurred in my immediate neighborhood. The disease made its appearance on the opposite side of the Missouri river, in Howard county, eight or ten miles below my residence.

No sooner was it ascertained that it was cholera, than the people fled to this side of the river, and encamped, panic-struck, as if an all-devouring demon had visited them. Dr. Penn and myself being the only physicians residing in this county at that time, they kept us most of the time with them; and we were, perhaps, as much alarmed as most of them: yet we encouraged them to be of good cheer, and not to be affrighted at what had happened.

About this time, bowel-complaints were unusually prevalent in this neighborhood. Our neighbors soon took fright, and came to us, hourly, for medicine and advice. Those who had not actual bowel-complaints, imagined they had something that was worse. A general panic and consternation now overspread the land.

We furnished them with laudanum and essence of peppermint; and, in case of an actual attack of cholera, informed them what to do, until one or the other of us should arrive. We also advised them to be cheerful; to follow their usual employments in moderation; to eat and drink as usual; except to be more sparing in the use of fresh meats, and raw and indigestible vegetables.

As many of them were almost frightened into real cholera, had we done as some other physicians did,—advise them to take to their beds, and commence the use of medicines,—many that were not sick, or who escaped the disease, in all probability would have taken it in reality.

The first case of cholera that I met with, convinced me, that if the disease was within the reach of medical treatment, it must consist, exclusively, of that class of medicines called restoratives; or such things as would arrest the progress of waste, and promptly recal and sustain the natural tonic action. For this purpose, I used large and repeated doses of laudanum; large and repeated draughts of strong, hot toddy; essence of pepper-mint; camphor, and red-pepper tea.

I prescribed stimulating frictions to the skin, in preference to warm bathing, and advised the patients to keep their beds. When the stools were frequent, and accompanied with pain, I administered laudanum, by injection. I directed a tea-spoonfull of laudanum to the gill of starch, or gruel; to be repeated as occasion required.

I have pointed out, in a summary way, what I conceive to be the indications of cure, and mentioned the remedies that I used to meet these indications with: I will now say something of their doses, and the circumstances under which they should be continued, moderated in their use, or entirely discontinued.

Cholera, taken in the premonitory stage, is a mild and manageable disease; but requires vigilance and prudence to prevent it from running into confirmed cholera. These symptoms are a mild looseness, with indigestion, and attended with little or no pain; of longer or shorter duration.—Commonly preceding an attack from one to three or four days. In this mild form, or stage of the disease, the patient should take from fifteen to twenty drops of laudanum, four or five times a day, to check, and to hold in check, this looseness of the bowels; they should, at the same time, be attentive to diet and to exercise, avoiding all imprudences and excesses.

But sometimes the attacks come on more violently, without giving any previous notice; so that, in an hour or two, the patient is completely prostrated, and the disease assumes all its characteristic features—such as the rice-water, and the milk-and-water-like discharges, either from stomach and bowels, or both, accompanied with partial or general spasm. In all such cases, I gave from sixty to eighty drops of laudanum, with fifteen or twenty drops of essence of pepper-mint, in a good portion of strong toddy; or, if the pepper-mint was not at hand, in its place I used a tea-spoonful of the tincture of camphor, or two or three table-spoonfuls of strong, red-pepper tea; sometimes, also, a tea-spoonful of the tincture of kino.

It should be always borne in mind, that if the dose of medicine is cast up by puking, it should be repeated so soon as the stomach becomes a little settled; because little or no benefit could result from it, unless it is retained.

It will not be considered an extravagant use of laudanum, or other articles, when it is recollected that a large portion of all the medicines taken run off by the bowels before they have time to act on the general system; and that when the evacuations are checked, that then we suspend the use of the remedies.

In cases of locked-jaw, and in some other violent spasmodic affections, it is a common practice to give as large, and even much larger doses of laudanum, than I have recommended in cholera. In such cases, too, the medicines are all retained,—not thrown off by the bowels,—and it is the article mainly relied on to counteract the spasm.

Laudanum is given in cholera not more with a view to allay the spasm and painful sensations, than to check the inordinate discharges from the stomach and bowels; the ultimate effect of which every medical man must know, however much he may be opposed to the practice of putting a sudden check to such discharges. The external frictions and injections, mentioned above, should be attended to as circumstances may require. With me, the first object is, to arrest the debilitating and exhausting discharges, and, at the same time, to allay pain, and to quiet and compose the general system. These objects accomplished, then much smaller doses of laudanum should be given; but it should not be entirely discontinued. This treatment should be kept up for two or three days, so as to restrain all action of the bowels. While the quantity of laudanum and kino is lessened, the free use of the toddy should be continued until the patient is considered out of danger.

So soon as all the violent symptoms have abated, and the system becomes composed, the patient should begin to take some very light diet, well seasoned—taking, however, but little at a time, and gradually increasing the quantity and changing the quality of the food to suit the strength of the patient. They should commence with such articles as tea, coffee, boiled milk, thickened milk, soups, and the like.

Until the year 1835, I had not seen consecutive fevers succeed cholera. That season the cholera broke out at Arrow Rock, a small town situated on the Missouri river, in Saline county, five miles distant from my residence. In that place and its vicinity sixteen or eighteen persons took it in its various degrees of intensity; and out of that number only one person died.

Dr. Price had the management of most of those cases, and I am much pleased to state that his treatment was very similar to that of Dr. Penn and my own, in 1833.

A few weeks after it appeared at Arrow Rock, it visited two families in my immediate neighborhood;—a few scattered cases besides occurred, fifteen of which ran into confirmed cholera; and each case was followed by more or less of consecutive fever. In some instances the cholera symptoms had scarcely ceased when the fever made its appearance. I treated this fever with sulphate of quinine, in grain doses, every two or three hours, until there was a complete crisis, or solution of diseased action—at the same time continuing the toddy and laudanum as circumstances seemed to require.

Whether it was from good fortune or from good treatment I know not, but my patients all recovered.

I did not find it necessary to give cathartic medicines after treating my cases with opiates and astringents; for, after the lapse of three or four days, the bowels always took a regular and healthy action of themselves, and without the patient's feeling the slightest fulness or uneasiness of any kind; and should the bowels have failed to take on natural action in due time, I would have preferred the use of mild injections to any cathartic drugs.

Strange as this practice may appear to many physicians, I am, nevertheless, confirmed in the belief of its correctness, not only from the success attending it in 1835, but also from the results of it in 1833, when Dr. Penn and myself attended 35 cases of regular and well marked cho-era. Of this number only two proved fatal, both of which were far advanced in the disease before we saw them.

The whole number of cases in the two years, that is, the two visitations of 1833 and 1835, were about 80 well marked cases; of this number we lost but three.

The same year that the cholera raged here it also raged at St. Louis, and in other parts of the State, with its usual fatality—under the common treatment of bleeding, puking, and purging. It was in St. Louis, Palmyra, Boonville, Chariton, and other places in the State, and from the best information that I could obtain, at least three-fourths, if not more of the cases proved fatal. Unless it was owing to the treatment, why should it be so much more fatal in all other sections of the State, and everywhere else, than it was under the treatment which I here recommend?

In my treatment of cholera I have never given one grain of calomel, or any other nauseating medicine. If any other mode of treatment has been more successful, I have not yet learned it. I know not from what cause cholera is produced, nor does it matter, in a practical point of view; be it what it may, I am decidedly of opinion that it should be treated with stimulants, opiates and astringents, throughout.

Consecutive fever is like other fevers, only that it has its beginning under circumstances of greater exhaustion and functional derangement, and must therefore require, necessarily, the use of tonics and stimulants from the commencement. These remedies have a tendency to correct fever, and to sustain exhausted and sinking nature.

In conclusion, I will briefly state that in 1833, the first year that I witnessed any cases of cholera, that as soon as the disease was evidently arrested, and warmth restored to the surface of the body, the patients all recovered more rapidly than in any other disease I had ever witnessed.— They seemed to have nothing but extreme debility to overcome; while in 1835, nearly half the cases were followed by consecutive fever, and in some instances the fever appeared at least as dangerous as the cholera itself; and all recovered from the fever rather slowly, though not more so than in other low cases of fever.

THE END.

CPSIA information can be obtained
at www.ICGtesting.com
Printed in the USA
LVOW04*0454080716
495600LV00009B/35/P